D1130713

JENNER'S
SMALLPOX
VACCINE

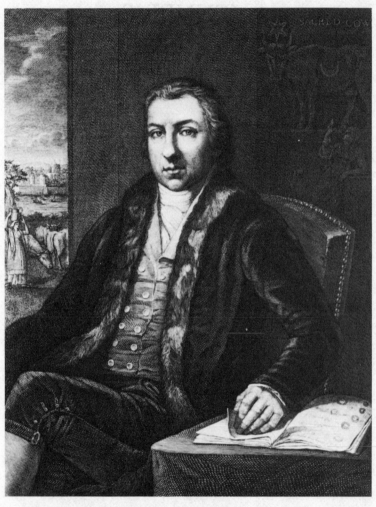

Frontispiece Edward Jenner by Monsaldi. The story behind this
unusual engraving is told in Baxby (1978). (Author's Collection.)

JENNER'S SMALLPOX VACCINE

The Riddle of Vaccinia Virus and its Origin

Derrick Baxby

Senior Lecturer in Medical Microbiology
University of Liverpool

Heinemann Educational Books

Published in Great Britain by
Heinemann Educational Books Ltd
22 Bedford Square, London WC1B 3HH

LONDON   EDINBURGH   MELBOURNE   AUCKLAND
HONG KONG   SINGAPORE   KUALA LUMPUR   NEW DELHI
IBADAN   NAIROBI   JOHANNESBURG   KINGSTON
EXETER (NH)   PORT OF SPAIN

ISBN 0 435 54057 2

First published 1981

For John and Anne

British Library Cataloguing in Publication Data

Baxby, Derrick
    Jenner's smallpox vaccine.
    1. Jenner, Edward
    2. Smallpox – Preventative – vaccination –
    History
    I. Title
    614.5'21   R489.J5
    ISBN 0-435-5407-2

Printed and bound in Great Britain by
Morrison & Gibb Ltd, London and Edinburgh

Contents

Foreword by Professor Frank Fenner   vi

Preface   ix

List of Illustrations   xii

Author's Note   xiii

1   The Riddle Outlined   1

2   Smallpox   10

3   Smallpox Prevention before Jenner   21

4   Edward Jenner   38

5   Jenner's *Inquiry*   52

6   Reactions to the *Inquiry*   70

7   The Jenner-Woodville Controversy   89

8   Ann Bumpus   105

9   Other Early Vaccines   118

10   True and Spurious Cowpox   134

11   Attenuation of Smallpox   150

12   Cowpox and Grease   165

13   The Origins of Vaccinia   179

Literature Cited   197

Index   210

Foreword

The certification of the eradication of smallpox from Africa was signalled by a ceremony in Nairobi on 26 October 1979, two years after recognition of the last case of endemic smallpox in Africa, and the world, in the town of Merka, in Somalia. On 8 May 1980, the World Health Assembly adopted a resolution which 'declared solemnly that the world and all its peoples have won freedom from smallpox. . .'. These two events marked an unprecedented event in human history; the deliberate worldwide eradication of an important human disease. This was the ultimate fulfilment of the prophecy made in 1801 by Dr Edward Jenner, and it was made possible, as Jenner foresaw, by the practice of vaccination.

Although variolation (the deliberate inoculation of small-pox virus) had considerably reduced the lethal impact of smallpox in many countries during the late eighteenth century, this practice was intrinsically incompatible with eradication, since it could, and did, produce unmodified smallpox in unprotected contacts. Jenner's great discovery was the use of an antigenically related virus that protected inoculated persons against smallpox but was not transmissible to contacts.

However, even now we do not know where vaccinia virus came from. Some years ago, when the idea of using latinized binomial nomenclature for viral species was in vogue, it was called *Poxvirus officinale*, but this name merely sidestepped the issue as to whether it originated from smallpox virus, cowpox virus, some other unspecified poxvirus, or by hybridization between such viruses. Analysis of the genetic material of several strains of smallpox, vaccinia, and cowpox viruses has confirmed their characterization as distinct viral species, already made by biological tests. The structure of their genomes is such that the 'transformation' of one species into another, a hypothesis previously advanced for the origin of vaccinia virus, is impossible. Indeed it is difficult to see how any one of these poxviruses could come exactly to resemble another even after many passages in a novel host and many sequential mutational changes.

In this book Dr Derrick Baxby, who has made a special study of the biological characteristics and natural history of members of the genus *Orthopoxvirus,* to which smallpox, cowpox, and vaccinia viruses belong, examines the biological nature of vaccinia virus and the historical evidence relating to its origin, from the time of Jenner up to the present day. Like other scientists who have studied this problem, he has been unable to reach a definitive conclusion, although several previously popular hypotheses have been shown to be wrong. Influenced by his own recent demonstration that cowpox virus is not what its name implies, primarily a disease of cows, but may be a disease of rodents which occasionally infects cows, man, and other mammals, Dr Baxby suggests that vaccinia virus may derive from a now extinct poxvirus disease of horses and possibly other animals, including small rodents. It is possible that investigations of viral diseases of wild rodents now being undertaken in Europe will provide evidence for this hypothesis; currently it must be regarded as unproven, but in developing his argument Dr Baxby does lay to rest several unsupportable hypotheses that had been advanced in the past.

Coming just at the time of the global eradication of smallpox, the book is timely. It gives proper credit to Jenner for his revolutionary demonstration, by experiment, that it was possible to protect humans against one viral disease by infecting them with a different but related virus, and it makes an important contribution to one of the conundrums of virology: what were the origins of vaccinia virus?

Frank Fenner
Chairman,
Global Commission for the
Certification of Smallpox
Eradication.

Preface

In 1979 the World Health Organization announced the total eradication of smallpox, a disease which in 1967 infected probably ten million people. The eradication campaign could not have succeeded without an efficient vaccine yet the actual origins of smallpox vaccine have, to quote Fritz Dekking, 'in spite of much endevour, remained an unsolved riddle of virology'. In this book I have attempted to solve that riddle by analysing the possible origins of the vaccines introduced by Edward Jenner and his contemporaries, and of the later vaccines, in the light of up-to-date information on the behaviour of smallpox, cowpox, and vaccinia viruses. Such an analysis has not been attempted before except briefly in my paper in the *Journal of the History of Medicine* on which this book is partly based. Because the subject is of general interest I have tried to make the virological and medical arguments intelligible to those with no specific knowledge of these topics and have included a general chapter on smallpox to provide necessary background information.

This book is not a biography of Jenner, nor an account of smallpox and its eradication, nor an account of the development of commercial vaccine, although information on these topics will be found here. Further information on these subjects may be obtained from the literature listed at the end of the book. In order to provide maximum information, without too long or complicated a system of references, I have included in the text where necessary the relevant page numbers of the books which are cited. In this way the need to use *op cit* and *ibid* references has been largely avoided. Much of the earlier literature on smallpox vaccination is rare and inaccessible. Consequently I have frequently quoted the actual words used by the early workers; in most cases the original words are better than any modern paraphrase, and in addition they help to evoke the character of the times in which they were written. All the italics in the quotations are as used by the original authors. I have also taken the opportunity to include important and inaccessible illustrations from the early literature, many of which have not been previously reproduced. Unfortunately the condition of some of the originals means that the quality of some of the illustrations is not as high as I would like.

I would like to thank the following who provided material for illustrations: The University of Liverpool for Figures 3, 6, 7, and 10; Liverpool Medical Institution for Figures 2, 5, 13, 14, and 21; Dr Paul Gibbs for Figures 17 and 20; Dr R. T. D. Emond for Figure 11. Figures 1 and 12 are reproduced by courtesy of the Trustees of the British Museum and of the Wellcome Historical Museum respectively. The remaining Figures are from my own collection.

The Frontispiece and Figures 10 and 15 have appeared previously in my papers in *Medical History* and *Journal of the History of Medicine*. Figures 9, 16, and 18 are reproduced with the permission of the Editor of the *British Medical Journal*, Figure 11 with the permission of Dr Emond and Wolfe Medical Publications, and Figures 17 and 20 with the permission of Dr Gibbs and the Editor of the *Veterinary Record*.

As a laboratory scientist I ventured into medical history with some trepidation and I would like to acknowledge the generous help and encouragement which I have received from William Le Fanu, Donald Henderson, Leonard Wilson, and particularly from Frank Fenner who kindly agreed to write the Foreword. My interest in many aspects of pox-virology has benefited from stimulating discussions over many years with Professors Kevin McCarthy and Allan Downie.

I would like to thank Mr D. M. Crook for generously allowing me to use the valuable material in the library of the Liverpool Medical Institution, and Mrs Margaret Kerr for typing the manuscript. Finally I would like to thank my wife for putting up with the many evenings which I spent submerged in paper, and also for her help with checking, indexing, and proof-reading.

List of Illustrations

Frontispiece   Edward Jenner, from an engraving by
Monsaldi   ii
1   *The Cow Pock,* caricature by James Gillray   7
2   Jenner's account of the variolation of William
   Stinchcomb   57
3   Accidental human cowpox 1796, Sarah Nelmes
   (Jenner)   58
4   Chart showing Jenner's vaccinations of 1796 and
   1798   59
5   Jenner's account of the vaccination of William
   Pead   60
6   William Pead's vaccination lesion (Jenner)   61
7   Hannah Excell's vaccination lesions (Jenner)   62
8   Accidental human cowpox, 1973   76
9   Accidental human cowpox, 1888 (Crookshank)   77
10   Vaccination and variolation compared, 1801
   (Paytherus)   81
11   Typical primary vaccination, 1974 (Emond)   84
12   William Woodville, from an engraving by Bond   90
13   Woodville's account of the vaccination of Ann
   Bumpus   92
14   Extract from the Table in Woodville's *Reports*   93
15   Pedigree of one of Woodville's vaccines   106
16   Clinical chart of smallpox, variolation, and vaccination, 1896 (Hime)   110
17   True and spurious cowpox, 1970 (Gibbs)   139
18   Accidental human cowpox, 1888 (Crookshank)   147
19   Accidental human cowpox, 1889 (Crookshank)   149
20   Bovine cowpox, 1970 (Gibbs)   172
21   Bovine cowpox, 1840 (Ceely)   173
22   Electronmicrograph of cowpox-infected cell   186

Author's Note

Before the introduction of smallpox vaccination, protection against naturally-occurring smallpox could be obtained by the deliberate inoculation of smallpox virus into the skin. This was simply called *inoculation* and until 1798 this term had no other medical meaning. When Jenner introduced his method of preventing smallpox by the inoculation of cowpox it was necessary to distinguish between the two methods. The original inoculation became known as *variolation* and this term will be used in this book. Jenner's method was variously referred to as cowpoxing, cowpox inoculation, vaccine inoculation, and vacciolation until the term *vaccination* became generally accepted. It is not known precisely when and by whom this term was originally introduced although it is usually attributed to Richard Dunning of Plymouth (Baron, 1838, II, p. 336).

The terms *vaccine* and *vaccination* were used only in connection with smallpox until 1881. However, in 1881 Pasteur proposed that they should be used to describe any prophylactic immunization. Although Pasteur intended to honour Jenner by this proposal it introduced a certain amount of confusion. It is now customary to talk of polio vaccine, measles vaccine, etc., and the terms vaccine and vaccination have lost their original specific meaning. In this book *vaccine* and *vaccination* are used in their original meaning and the qualifying term 'smallpox' is frequently omitted.

The early vaccinators, particularly Jenner, used the word *virus* in a way which seems very natural to modern readers. However, by their use of this word, the early workers were simply referring to a *specific transmissible poison*, the nature of which was a mystery. They had no idea that particulate infective agents, now called viruses, were responsible. This dual meaning should be remembered in those chapters where the behaviour of early vaccine viruses is analysed in the light of up-to-date information on smallpox and related viruses.

I

The Riddle Outlined

Most people will associate the name of Edward Jenner with smallpox vaccination. Many credit Jenner with the introduction of vaccination in 1796, some think that he has been given too much credit, and a few deny him any credit at all. Although smallpox vaccination was accepted quickly, not just in England but also abroad, it aroused considerable controversy from the very beginning. Basically there were three sources of argument.

The principal one, of course, was whether vaccination really offered any protection against smallpox. The original idea that vaccination offered life-long protection was soon found to be incorrect. However, the evidence that vaccination, properly carried out, will reduce the incidence of smallpox is so strong that it need not be considered in detail in this book, although some references will be made to it. For vaccination to have any effect at all it was essential that the vaccine contained the correct active agent – a virus immunologically related to smallpox virus. Vaccination was introduced approximately 100 years before the existence of viruses was demonstrated and many arguments raged which concerned the effects of 'true' and 'spurious' cowpox vaccines; these will be discussed in Chapter 10. The second argument concerned the safety of vaccination and the possibility that other diseases, particularly syphilis, were transmitted by vaccination. This is really a consequence of the fact that vaccination was developed as an empirical procedure without any real knowledge of how its production and quality could be controlled, and this problem will not be discussed here. It was to be almost 100 years before Pasteur introduced the next vaccines against rabies, anthrax, and chicken cholera.

The third question is the one which this book examines in some detail. What was the identity of the viruses in the earliest vaccines and to whom should credit be given for their introduction? No certain answer can be given. The evidence has been analysed many times with no great agreement. This book attempts to provide, not so much a definite answer, as an objective survey which examines the various alternatives presented by the historical record in the light of present-day virological knowledge. An easier question to answer is: Why should there be doubt about the identity of the vaccines introduced so long ago? – everyone knows that Jenner used cowpox to induce immunity to smallpox. Certainly it has been generally accepted that Jenner used cowpox although some have reservations which will be discussed later. During Jenner's time there was debate as to whether cowpox was a separate disease or simply smallpox virus infection of the cow. Consequently the earliest alternatives for the identity of the vaccine virus were that it was either cowpox or a modified form of smallpox, attenuated by passage through the cow.

Smallpox virus is a member of the genus *Orthopoxvirus*. Other members of this genus include cowpox, vaccinia, monkeypox, camelpox, and buffalopox (Baxby, 1975). The viruses are all closely related and the interrelationships of smallpox, cowpox, and vaccinia viruses will be discussed in later chapters. The particular characteristic which unites all members of the genus is that infection with one member will confer specific immunity to the other members.

The vaccines originally introduced were gradually replaced during the nineteenth century and the only information we have concerning their identity comes from the engravings and printed descriptions. Some confusion is caused by the fact that different early vaccines gave slightly different effects. It is not known whether this was due to differences in the identity of the virus or to contaminating bacteria.

However, the major source of doubt is the fact that strains of cowpox virus, isolated in recent years, are quite different from the many strains of vaccine (i.e. vaccinia virus) which have been examined. This difference was first demonstrated in 1939 by A. W. Downie. Although some American workers continued to use the terms cowpox and vaccinia synonymously for a number of years, the fact that they are different has been confirmed and is now generally accepted.

Cowpox is found only in Britain and Western Europe, and was so named because it was isolated from cattle and from farmworkers in contact with them. Until recently it was believed that the virus was enzootic in cattle, i.e. that cows were its natural reservoir. However, bovine cowpox is rare and human cases occur without any contact with bovine infection. Consequently it is now believed that both cattle and humans become infected accidentally and that the reservoir is some, as yet unidentified, small wild mammal (Baxby, 1977a, b). Bovine cowpox has always been relatively rare and we know that Jenner and the earlier vaccinators sometimes had difficulty in obtaining supplies. Consequently we might wonder whether 'cowpox', as we know it, was enzootic in cattle at that time. This is something which will be discussed more fully in Chapter 12.

In contrast to all other poxviruses vaccinia has no natural reservoir. It is maintained in laboratories for research purposes and for smallpox vaccine production. It has been isolated from a number of animal species including cows, camels, buffaloes, and pigs, but the source of infection has been a recently vaccinated person and the virus has not become established in the animal species. From this reasonable and generally accepted view that vaccinia virus is not now found naturally, has grown the belief that it never occurred naturally and that it could not have been used by the original vaccinators. Consequently, various alternative explanations have been put forward to explain the origins of vaccinia virus. Before 1939 the argument simply was whether 'vaccine' (then assumed to be the same as cowpox) was derived from smallpox or was a separate animal poxvirus. Since 1939 theories have had to account for the now separate identities of vaccinia and cowpox. The various theories can be briefly listed.

1. That vaccinia has been derived from cowpox by repeated passage in vaccine institutions. The main proponent of this theory is A. W. Downie. However, this origin assumes that the early vaccines really were cowpox, an assumption which will be examined in detail later.

2. The development of vaccinia by the adaptation of smallpox virus to growth in animals had some strong advocates in England and Germany up to the end of the 1930s. These claims were based on early experimental approaches which were not always well controlled, and the theory finds little support at the present time. One of the last reported transformations of smallpox into vaccinia was made in 1938 by E. S. Horgan.

3. Also strongly advocated in the nineteenth century was the view that vaccinia had been derived from smallpox by serial arm-to-arm transfer in humans. This method of propagating vaccine was used in the first half of the century until gradually replaced by the use of vaccine prepared on the skin of cows or sheep. This theory has recently had a revival through the writings of P. E. Razzell.

4. An attractive theory proposed in the 1960s by K. R. Dumbell and H. S. Bedson is that vaccinia evolved as a genetic hybrid between smallpox and cowpox viruses. Such hybridization could have occurred when people were vaccinated with contaminated vaccine or even when vaccinated with vaccine to which smallpox virus had been deliberately added.

5. The fact that vaccinia does not exist naturally now, does not necessarily mean that it never had a natural reservoir. However, the possibility that the original vaccinators might have actually used a virus which we would recognize as vaccinia has received little attention until my own recent inquiries.

It is unfortunate that most previous writers, particularly in the nineteenth century, dogmatically advocated a single origin. Perhaps they thought that the strength of the argument in support of their favourite origin would be reduced if they admitted that an occasional vaccine may have had a different origin. However, we know that not all early vaccines produced the same results and this might be due to their containing different viruses. In addition the many modern strains of vaccinia differ in their laboratory characteristics and human pathogenicity. This again may be a reflection of different origins. It would be surprising if all the many vaccines which have been introduced during the past 180 years had the same origin.

Although Jenner introduced vaccination to the public the actual evidence on which his claims were based was very limited and his vaccine strains were not widely used. The first extensive trials of vaccination were carried out in 1799 by William Woodville, Director of the London Smallpox and Inoculation Hospital. Although Woodville started with vaccine material obtained from a cow, he carried out his trials in the Smallpox Hospital. His results differed from Jenner's in that approximately 2/3 of his cases developed smallpox and it is generally agreed that they became infected with smallpox at about the time they were vaccinated. There is still doubt about how they contracted smallpox and continuing doubt about the identity of Woodville's vaccines. Woodville collaborated with George Pearson, a physician of St George's Hospital, and they distributed their vaccine widely, not only in Britain but also abroad. Since these vaccines were used so widely their identity is crucial to the problem of the origins of vaccinia and to whether the most credit is due to Jenner or Woodville.

The problem has been analysed many times, sometimes in isolation, sometimes together with more practical investigations into the safety and effectiveness of vaccination. Some critics had very pertinent points to make on these issues, but some approaches were frankly hysterical. These last included some which maintained that vaccination was immoral and contrary to the will of God. This was at a time when it was firmly believed that Man had been created in God's own image, and some claimed that the inoculation of material from the 'brute animal' would impart bovine characteristics to the recipients. This was satirized in the famous print by James Gillray which shows cows erupting from the various lesions produced by the vaccine which had been obtained 'hot from ye cow'.

Parliament debated vaccination in 1802 in connection with Jenner's claim for recognition. They heard evidence from both his supporters and opponents. These latter included those who opposed both vaccination and Jenner, and others like George Pearson, who supported vaccination, but sought recognition for themselves. Parliament found in Jenner's favour (*see* George Jenner, 1805). In 1857 Sir John Simon prepared a report on vaccination for the General Board of Health, which was also presented to Parliament (Simon, 1857). This again found in Jenner's favour and attested to the safety and effectiveness of vaccination.

These investigations reached a peak in the last two decades of the nineteenth century. During this period serious epidemics of smallpox in England had led to the setting up of a Royal Commission on Vaccination in 1889, and the publication of its summary report in 1898 coincided with the centenary of the publication of Jenner's *Inquiry*. Although the Royal Commission was primarily concerned with the effectiveness and safety of vaccination it also considered evidence relating to the origin of vaccinia. The verdict of the majority of the Commissioners was again in Jenner's favour. They decided that his early investigations although limited were sufficiently sound. As regards Woodville's practice they decided that although most of his patients did have smallpox, the vaccines which emerged and which were widely distributed were not derived from smallpox (Royal Commission, 1898). This view was also taken by John C. McVail writing in the Jenner Centenary Issue of the *British Medical Journal*

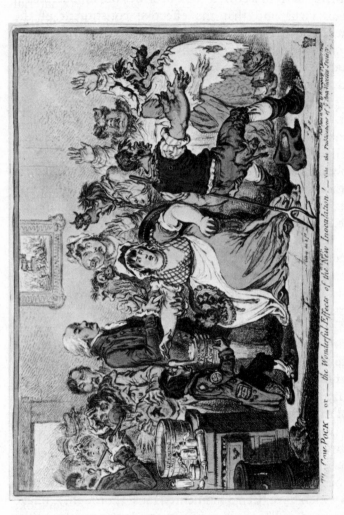

Figure 1 The Cow Pock by James Gillray. Edward Jenner is usually said to be the central figure of this famous caricature. However Abraham, in his biography of Lettsom, (1933, p.351) suggested that the central character was George Pearson. (Reproduced by Courtesy of the Trustees of the British Museum).

(McVail, 1896). However, a minority of the Royal Commissioners took a contrary view and appended a Dissentient Report. They believed that although Woodville started off by using material from a cow, it soon became contaminated with smallpox virus and that the effective constituent of the vaccines, which became so widely distributed, was attenuated smallpox (Royal Commission, 1898). In this view vaccination was nothing more than an extension of the procedure of inoculating the smallpox (*variolation*), first tested in England in 1721, and so no credit at all was due to Jenner. Particularly strong holders of this view were Edgar M. Crookshank (1889) and Charles Creighton (1889). Creighton believed most strongly that Jenner had perpetrated an enormous hoax on society in general and on the medical profession in particular, and as we shall see this led to him holding views on Jenner which were almost mutually exclusive. There was also some inconsistency in Crookshank's views. The idea that Woodville's vaccines were attenuated smallpox and that no credit is due to Jenner has been revived in recent years by Peter Razzell (1965, 1977). Although his analyses failed to take account of other alternatives, equally valid as an origin from smallpox, he did call for more investigation into the subject.

In this book I have examined the events surrounding the introduction and development of the earliest smallpox vaccines and, making use of present-day virological information, have tried to interpret these events in the light of each of the various theories for the origin of vaccinia. Apart from my recent paper, on which this book is based (Baxby, 1979), this is the first time this has been attempted.

It has been rightly said that the origins of vaccinia will never be known. The closest we can come is to examine those events which have been documented most thoroughly. I have concentrated on Woodville's practice and in particular on the possible origins of a strain of vaccine which he derived from a patient named Ann Bumpus. This particular strain was sent to Jenner and some believe that it was not only representative of Woodville's vaccines but also that it was distributed widely. As will be discussed here these assumptions are not necessarily valid. Nevertheless, the Bumpus strain has always received a lot of attention, and rightly or wrongly the origin of this strain has always been considered as central to the problem of the origins of vaccinia in general and to the claims of Jenner's supporters that he be given the most credit for the introduction of vaccination.

These events have been placed in perspective by briefly considering the importance of smallpox and attempts made to prevent it before the Jennerian era, by describing the introduction of other early vaccines, and by discussing the later attempts which were made to develop vaccines from smallpox virus.

2

Smallpox

In October 1977, in Merka village near Mogadishu, the capital of Somalia, a twenty-three-year-old cook caught smallpox. It is extremely likely that this will be the last case of naturally-acquired smallpox anywhere in the world.

In 1967 the World Health Organization set up a unit headed by Donald A. Henderson whose task was the total eradication of smallpox. In 1967, 44 countries reported a total of 131,418 cases of smallpox, but because of poor surveillance and reporting at the start of the campaign, Henderson (1976a) estimated that the actual number of cases was probably closer to ten million. The principal areas affected were India, Pakistan, and Bangladesh, the Indonesian archipelago, Africa south of the Sahara, and Brazil. The last case of smallpox in Brazil occurred in 1971 and in Indonesia in 1972. Eradication in the Indian subcontinent and parts of Africa was hindered by civil unrest, but the last case in Asia was reported from Bangladesh in 1975. Experience had shown that an area could be declared free of smallpox if no cases occurred in the two years following the last known case. This required extensive searches often in very remote areas, not only to seek out missed indigenous cases but also imported cases. As an example of the thoroughness of the searches we can take that of India and Bangladesh quoted by Henderson's successor as chief of the Smallpox Eradication Unit, I. Arita. In the two years following the last case extensive house-to-house searches were made, three in India and eight in Bangladesh. It was calculated that each search covered 98 per cent of the 726,811 towns and villages in the two countries (Arita, 1979).

The eradication of smallpox from the Indian subcontinent is particularly significant. Not only was the incidence in that area very high, but the type of smallpox found there was the most virulent type (*variola major*) which could kill up to 60 per cent of those infected.

No more cases were detected in Somalia and the world was declared free of smallpox in October 1979. This is the first instance in which a human disease has been eradicated, and is a remarkable monument to international co-operation and the practice of preventive medicine.

There are a number of features which combine to make smallpox an almost unique candidate for eradication. For the present we need only consider the fact that it is an easily recognized serious disease which has threatened man for centuries. The success of the Smallpox Eradication Campaign, and before it the local successes which eliminated smallpox from Europe and North America have resulted in populations with little idea of the impact which smallpox made on previous generations. Only the briefest account can be given here. Those particularly interested should consult C. W. Dixon's *Smallpox* (1962) and Frank Fenner's *Smallpox and its Eradication* (in press) for more information. Donald G. Hopkins of Atlanta, Georgia, has collected a lot of hitherto unpublished data on the history of smallpox which it is hoped will be published soon.

The origins of smallpox are not known with certainty, and the further back one looks the less is the certainty that the disease being described really was smallpox. It is believed to have existed in India and China for thousands of years, and the mummified head of Rameses V, who died in 1160 B.C., is thought to show the characteristic pocks of the disease. However, no disease recognizable as smallpox is described in either the writings of classical Greece and Rome or in the Bible. The first clear account of smallpox is probably that by the Persian physician Rhazes in about A.D. 900 (Rhazes, 1848). Smallpox was probably established in Europe as a result of the Moorish conquest of Spain and by Crusaders returning from the Holy Land. It was apparently unknown in the Americas until introduced by the Spanish invaders who followed in the wake of Columbus.

During the seventeenth and eighteenth centuries smallpox began to have a definite, recorded impact on Western society. This impact can be measured in various ways and only a few examples can be given. It has been estimated that the smallpox deaths in Europe during the eighteenth century numbered 200,000–600,000 each year. If the deaths from smallpox in England during this period are corrected for the increase in population they would be equivalent to over 100,000 deaths from smallpox each year in the 1970s. Similar numbers of deaths are now being caused by heart disease or cancer. However, whereas these diseases kill mainly adults, smallpox killed mainly children. Deaths from smallpox accounted for 1/8–1/14 of all deaths, and could account for 1/3 of deaths in young children. Estimates of smallpox deaths were probably more accurate than estimates of the total incidence since mild cases would often go unrecorded. However, an overall estimate that 1/5–1/8 of smallpox patients died is generally accepted, although in some epidemics the mortality would be 50 per cent or higher. As an example of a typical epidemic in an English town we can take that in Chester in 1774, investigated by John Haygarth. The population was 14,713 and there were 1,202 cases of smallpox with 202 deaths. Thus about 1/12 of the population were infected and 1/6 of those died. All those dying were children. The fact that only 1/12 of the population caught smallpox is due to the fact that almost everyone else had had it in previous epidemics for Haygarth found that only 1/15 of the population had not previously had smallpox.

Emphasis has rightly been placed on the mortality, but it should be remembered that the survivors were very often badly disfigured and that smallpox was a major cause of blindness.

The impact of smallpox can also be measured by its effect

on the Royal houses of Europe. The effect on the English Royal Family following the restoration of Charles II in 1660 is a case in point. In 1660 Henry, Duke of Gloucester, and Princess Mary both died of smallpox. They were brother and sister of Charles II. Princess Mary's husband, William of Orange, had died of smallpox in 1650. Their son, William III of England, had smallpox and his wife Queen Mary, daughter of James II and niece of Charles II, died of smallpox in 1694. William's successor Anne had a bad attack but survived, but the death from smallpox of her last-surviving son in 1700 brought the crisis over the succession to a head and precipitated the Act of Settlement of 1701. It is not surprising that Caroline of Ansbach, wife of the future George II, took such an interest in the attempts to prevent smallpox by variolation (*see* Chapter 3).

The impact of smallpox on virgin populations was particularly severe. It was first introducd into the Americas by Spanish Conquistadors. The success of Cortez in so quickly subjugating the Aztec civilization of Mexico with only about 500 men was certainly helped by the effect of smallpox on the Aztecs. It is estimated that $3\frac{1}{2}$ million died. The effect of smallpox on the North American Indians was equally devastating, as told by Stearn and Stearn (1945). In 1841 Catlin wrote 'Thirty millions of white men are now scuffling over the bodies and ashes of twelve millions of red men, six millions of whom have fallen to the smallpox' (quoted by Simon, 1857, pp. iii–iv). In most cases the infection was transmitted accidentally to the Indians, but there were certain instances when the infection was introduced via deliberately contaminated blankets.

We cannot assess the impact of smallpox in earlier centuries without making some comparison with other diseases. During the eighteenth century the only endemic infectious diseases in England with a higher death rate than smallpox were consumption (tuberculosis), and 'fevers', which included typhus, typhoid, and scarlet fever. Plague was a special case. It was calculated that it caused 68,596 deaths during the Great Plague in London in 1665, but Paul (1964) suggests that 100,000 might be a more realistic figure. However, in contrast to the ever-present smallpox, plague was a rare visitor. England remained free of plague from 1666 to 1909. The fear of smallpox is still best expressed in Macaulay's often-quoted words.

> That disease . . . was the most terrible of all the ministers of death. The havoc of the Plague has been far more rapid, but the Plague has visited our shores only once or twice within living memory; and the smallpox was always present, filling the churchyard with corpses, tormenting with constant fears all whom it had not yet stricken, leaving on those whose lives it spared the hideous traces of its power, turning the babe into a changeling at which the mother shuddered, and making the eyes and cheeks of the betrothed maiden objects of horror to the lover.

The extent to which smallpox was controlled by variolation will be examined briefly in Chapter 3. Even after the introduction of vaccination, smallpox epidemics continued. In general, however, the disease was most severe in the unvaccinated, and cases in the vaccinated tended to occur in adults whose immunity had begun to wane. For example, there was a serious epidemic in Sheffield in 1887–8, in which there were 6,088 cases with 590 deaths. The incidence in vaccinated children under 10 years was 5 per 1,000 and in the unvaccinated 101 per 1,000. The overall death rate was 11 per 1,000 in the vaccinated and 372 per 1,000 in the unvaccinated (Barry, 1889). There had been particularly severe epidemics in England in 1837–40, and 1870. The first of these, in which 42,000 died, led directly to the Vaccination Act of 1840 which outlawed variolation and provided free vaccination.

Although smallpox was endemic in Britain in the seventeenth to the nineteenth centuries the distribution of the population meant that some rural localities remained free for many years. Nor should it be thought that smallpox main-

tained the same virulence during this period. Different localized epidemics within a general endemic area often produced
mortalities higher or lower than the average figures quoted.

During the twentieth century the virulent form of smallpox
(variola major) persisted in Asia and parts of Africa and was
occasionally imported into Europe and America. However, a
much less virulent form with a mortality of one per cent or
less appeared in South Africa and became established in
Britain and the Americas. This was *alastrim* or *variola minor*.
In Britain during 1926–30 over 10,000 cases were reported
annually, but alastrim was then gradually eliminated. In the
United States over 35,000 cases were recorded annually in
1926–30 and over 10,000 cases annually up to 1939. It was
then controlled during the 1940s although occasional importations from Mexico continued to occur.

There have been occasional importations of variola major
into Britain and America since the Second World War
resulting in small epidemics which have usually been quickly
controlled. For example in England there were outbreaks on
Merseyside in 1946 which killed 14 out of 56 and in Brighton
in 1951 which killed 10 out of 37. Both these epidemics were
started by servicemen returning from overseas. Servicemen
returning to America in 1946 imported smallpox into Seattle
and California killing 28 out of 96.

The effect of these importations is not just measured in
terms of those killed or infected, tragic though they may be,
but also in terms of social and economic disruption. There
may be indiscriminate demands by a frightened population
for vaccination which will strain health services and lead to
further unnecessary deaths. For example in 1961–2 there were
6 separate importations of smallpox into England and Wales
resulting in at least 24 deaths out of 99 cases. There were
widespread demands for vaccination and $5\frac{1}{2}$ million doses of
vaccine were issued in 6 weeks. Many people were vaccinated
who were in no danger from smallpox, and for whom
vaccination itself was a danger, and Dick (1971) estimated
that at least 18 people died from complications of vaccination.

As the world incidence of smallpox decreased it was argued that there was greater danger in some countries from vaccination than from smallpox and in 1971 the United States and Britain ceased to recommend routine smallpox vaccination for children.

Tragic smallpox deaths have occurred recently in England, two in 1973 and one in 1978. In each instance the first person infected worked in a laboratory. However, it must not be thought from this that smallpox virus is particularly dangerous to handle. These tragedies occurred because a simple but essential administrative precaution was ignored. This is that no one should be allowed near a smallpox laboratory unless they have been properly vaccinated. Until 1973 it was considered safe for adequately vaccinated laboratory workers to deal with large quantities of smallpox virus on the open bench, and no case of smallpox has ever been reported in properly vaccinated laboratory workers. This, and the many physicians and nurses who have handled smallpox patients safely, is probably the most telling evidence of the effectiveness of vaccination. At the same time these tragedies and the unnecessary deaths of unvaccinated medical personnal is the most telling evidence of the need for proper vaccination.

As with the preceding historical account, only the briefest account can be given of clinical smallpox. *The Diagnosis of Smallpox*, by Ricketts and Byles (1908), is profusely illustrated and rightly considered a classic, but because of its narrow subject range is probably less useful than Dixon's *Smallpox* (1962), also profusely illustrated, which deals with all aspects of the disease. For shorter but still most authoritative accounts one should consult one of the chapters on smallpox contributed to a number of standard textbooks by Allan W. Downie of Liverpool.

Smallpox is an acute, infectious disease characterized by the development of a pustular eruption. Infection is via the upper respiratory tract, and during the incubation period of usually twelve days the virus spreads to and multiplies in the internal organs. At the end of the incubation period large numbers of virus particles are released into the bloodstream and this coincides with the first obvious signs of illness: fever, head- and back-ache, and prostration. This initial illness is not restricted to smallpox and may easily be confused with influenza or the early stages of typhoid. This pre-eruptive phase lasts from three to five days and then the characteristic rash develops. This appears first on the face, forearms, and hands and then spreads to the lower limbs and trunk. The eruption in smallpox is characteristically centrifugal; i.e. the lesions are more numerous on the face, hands, and forearms than on the upper arms and more numerous on the feet and calves than on the thighs and trunk. This is an important feature in distinguishing between smallpox and chickenpox where the eruption is more prominent on the trunk. In chickenpox the pre-eruptive illness is mild or absent and lesions can be found in different stages of development, whereas in smallpox, at any one time, they tend to be at the same stage. The lesions start as macules and progress through raised papules to vesicles filled with clear straw-coloured liquid. As the vesicles develop there is usually a drop in the patient's temperature. The vesicles become pustules and begin to dry to form crusts; crusting is usually complete about two weeks from the start of the illness. The crusts become separated by about three weeks. In any individual case the clinical picture may differ considerably from the above 'typical' account, and attempts have been made to classify different types of response based on severity. These vary from haemorrhagic smallpox which is invariably and rapidly fatal, through types of lesser severity with fewer lesions and a greater chance of survival. Smallpox in the vaccinated is usually less severe than in the unvaccinated, and may result in very few lesions and a very mild illness. Such a missed case has often proved an important source of infection. As the incubation period is about twelve days and immunity starts to develop about six to seven days after vaccination, then vaccination during the first week of the incubation period will often abort the infection or reduce its severity. Since 1963 a drug has been available (Marboran or Methisazone) which if given in the incubation period may prevent smallpox developing. The initial trials in Madras were extremely promising (Bauer *et al.*, 1969), and it is ironic that its development came at a time when the worldwide incidence of smallpox was being drastically reduced by the eradication campaign. Nothing is known which will cure smallpox once the illness has started.

Clinical differentiation between smallpox and chickenpox is not always easy. Confirmation can be obtained from the virus laboratory. Examination of vesicle fluid in the electron microscope will differentiate a poxvirus from the morphologically distinct herpesvirus which causes chickenpox. However, since smallpox virus is morphologically indistinguishable from the viruses of cowpox, monkeypox and vaccinia and these other viruses can occasionally produce a generalized infection like smallpox, the final diagnosis is made by differential biological tests. These usually include the characteristic appearance of the pocks produced on the chorioallantoic membrane surrounding the developing chick embryo, and suppression of these pocks by incubating the embryos at particular temperatures (Baxby, 1975). The key to successful smallpox control is the isolation of infected patients and the tracing, isolation, and vaccination of all contacts. Mass vaccination progammes had some success in reducing the total incidence of smallpox in endemic areas. However, following the campaign supervised in Nigeria by William H. Foege, emphasis has been placed on surveillance and vaccination of those at risk. This approach was shown to restrict and then eliminate foci of smallpox very efficiently (Foege *et al.*, 1975; Henderson, 1976b).

It might be useful to list those features which combine to make smallpox such a good candidate for eradication. As mentioned before it is a serious, easily recognized disease. Despite claims to the contrary it is not very communicable; although contaminated bedding or clothing may occasionally spread infection to laundry workers, infection is usually spread to only very close contacts. This, and the long incubation period, means that epidemics develop slowly, thus enabling control measures to be instigated. This is helped by the fact that patients are not infectious until the eruption develops; by this time they will be ill and their mobility will be reduced. There is no carrier state, unlike chickenpox where after a childhood infection the virus remains dormant in the nerve cells and may re-emerge many years later as shingles and start off a chickenpox epidemic in the next generation of children. Smallpox is believed to be an exclusively human disease; consequently eradication of smallpox in humans means total eradication with no reintroduction from an animal reservoir. Finally although strains of smallpox virus differ in virulence they are immunologically homogeneous and stable; consequently one vaccine introduced in 1796 will still serve in all cases.

The efficacy of vaccination need not be considered in detail here. Although opinions as to its efficacy have differed since its initial introduction it is clear that, properly used, it is very effective. However, it does not offer lifelong immunity. Estimates of the duration of immunity vary but obviously it is not an all-or-nothing phenomenon; the immunity will fall gradually with time. The WHO international vaccination certificate, which obviously errs on the side of safety, is valid for three years. However, it is evident that some degree of protection will be effective much longer than this.

The effectiveness of vaccination in protecting laboratory workers, physicians, and nurses has been mentioned. As an example of its value to the population in an endemic area we can use the observations made by A. R. Rao in Madras from 1961 to 1967. Of smallpox in the unvaccinated, 83 per cent of the cases were in children under 14 years old. In the vaccinated only 13 per cent of the cases were in children under 14 and the severity of infection was less (WHO, 1972). These figures show the protection afforded to young children by vaccination, and the need for re-vaccination to reinforce the immunity of young adults.

Of the factors just discussed, the possible origins of the vaccine used is the main subject of this book. Two others, the low communicability of smallpox and the absence of an animal reservoir are important when considering the possible derivation of vaccine from smallpox.

However, before examining these origins in detail, we must briefly examine attempts to control smallpox before the introduction of vaccination.

3

Smallpox Prevention before Jenner

As I have indicated already it was possible to obtain immunity from smallpox by *variolation* – the deliberate inoculation of smallpox virus into the skin under controlled conditions. It was hoped that this would produce a mild attack which would protect against a subsequent attack of natural small-pox which might have been more severe. As one possible origin of vaccinia virus is from smallpox virus by attenuation, some discussion of the effects of variolation is essential, particularly to assess any evidence that smallpox was becoming so attenuated by variolation as to resemble vaccinia. However, only a brief account need be given of its intro-duction into Western civilization. Authoritative accounts of its introduction into England and America have been given by Genevieve Miller (1957) and Ola Winslow (1974) respectively and Dixon has a brief but very readable account of variolation in general in his *Smallpox* (1962, pp. 216–48).

Information about variolation was obtained in the American colonies from Negro slaves in the first decade of the eighteenth century. At this time smallpox was not yet endemic in America, but epidemics were occasionally started from cases introduced from Europe. One person who was determ-ined to try variolation when the opportunity arose was the Rev. Cotton Mather, the first American-born Fellow of the Royal Society. His opportunity came in 1721 when he persuaded Dr Zabdiel Boylston to perform the first vario-lations in America.

Some discussions about the prevention of smallpox in China took place in the Royal Society from about 1700 onwards. However, the Chinese method was not strictly variolation. Instead of inoculating the virus into the skin, crusts containing the virus were inserted into the nostrils. Accounts of variolation were sent to the Royal Society in 1714 by Timoni of Athens and in 1716 by Pylarini, a Venetian. They described how in Turkey a mild form of the disease could be produced by inserting the virus into the skin. The first English people known to have been variolated, the sons of the secretary of the Ambassador to Turkey, arrived back in England in 1716.

The person whose name is always linked with the introduction of variolation into Britain is Lady Mary Wortley Montagu, although Genevieve Miller suggested that her influence has been over-emphasized. Lady Mary, the wife of the British Ambassador to Turkey, arrived in Constantinople in 1717. How much she knew of variolation before she left England is not clear, but within two weeks of reaching Constantinople she had written an enthusiastic letter to her friend Sarah Chiswell describing variolation. In the letter she announced her intention of introducing the practice into England. In 1717 she had her son successfully variolated in Constantinople. She returned to England in 1718. During the smallpox epidemic in London in 1721 she had her four-year-old daughter variolated by Charles Maitland who had been surgeon to the Embassy in Constantinople. Although evidence was soon forthcoming that variolation had been practised in remote regions of Wales and Scotland, this can be regarded as the first authenticated variolation in Britain.

Following this first variolation a trial was organized on six inmates of Newgate Prison who were promised freedom in exchange for their co-operation. The trials were conducted by Maitland, and observed by an eminent gathering of physicians and surgeons led by Sir Hans Sloane, physician to George I and President of the Royal Society. Five of the six had a mild smallpox, the sixth prisoner, who it was thought might have had smallpox some years before, was unaffected. The results of this trial were published by Maitland and reproduced by Dixon (1962, pp. 227–32), who described them as the first planned experiment in immunology. However, as such it merely demonstrated that smallpox could be transmitted by inoculation. Too few subjects were used to enable one to determine whether the effects would be consistently mild, and no attempt was made to determine, by subsequent re-variolation, whether they had developed any immunity. Nevertheless it was a start.

The next notable event, in 1723, was the successful variolation of the two children of Caroline of Ansbach, Princess of Wales, and the six children of Lord Bathurst. This might have been expected to provide a considerable boost to the practice. However, a footman who had been variolated at the same time died from smallpox. Although it cannot be determined whether he was killed by the inoculated virus, or by natural infection acquired whilst attending the variolated children, the damage had been done. There was considerable opposition to variolation, some of it reasonable but some of it, as with vaccination 70 years later, hysterical.

Variolation was not attempted to any great extent until the 1750s. Some have claimed that this was due to opposition to the practice, and that interest was renewed by safer methods introduced by the American variolator James Kirkpatrick. However, Genevieve Miller has pointed out that this fallacy was due to Kirkpatrick's talent for self-advertisement; she argued that the demand for variolation was high only during smallpox epidemics and that these were few from the 1720s to the 1740s (Miller, 1957, pp. 134–46). Another factor was the expense involved caused by a two- to four-week preparatory period before variolation and a similar convalescence after. Consequently variolation was only accepted by the well-to-do, and then only when necessary. In any event variolation became much more common from the 1750s onward when improved methods and plans for variolating the poor were introduced. It continued, still against some opposition, until the introduction of vaccination started a new controversy. In support of his view that vaccination was really an accidental and unrecognized attenuation of small-pox Razzell suggested that there was sufficient evidence that such attenuation was happening before the Jennerian period (Razzell, 1977a, b). Vaccination differed from variolation in three respects: (1) It was safe for the recipient; (2) It did not transmit infection to contacts; (3) There was no generalized eruption.

We can now briefly review variolation, in the light of present-day information on smallpox, to see whether there was any evidence that variolation led to the emergence of strains resembling vaccinia before vaccination was formally introduced.

Unfortunately there is little information about variolation in recent times which will serve as a source of comparison. Rosenwald in 1951 obtained first-hand information about variolation in Tanganyika. He observed that the majority of cases had mild smallpox although he saw one patient die and heard of others. He reported that in 'some cases' there was no generalized eruption, but that in others who apparently had just the lesion of inoculation he found vesicles on close examination. He was uncertain of the effect of variolation on the epidemic. He 'had the impression' that it helped to control the local epidemic but believed that it had helped to spread it to other localities.

There is no doubt that from the introduction of variolation into the Western world its mortality was much lower than that from natural smallpox. However, when estimating the number of deaths in variolated patients it is impossible to determine how many died from smallpox naturally acquired at the time they were being inoculated. As mentioned earlier 1/5–1/8 of smallpox patients died and in some epidemics this figure could rise to 1/2. Various estimates were made of the mortality from variolation in the early years, and there is some agreement on a figure of 1/50–1/70. The figures collected by the Royal Society for 1721–8 indicated 17 deaths in 858 successful variolations, a mortality of about 1/50 (Miller, 1957, p. 121). Woodville collected data in his *History of the Inoculation of the Smallpox in Great Britain* (1796). His figures for Boston, Mass., up to 1753 were 30 deaths out of 2,114, a mortality of about 1/70 (*ibid.*, p. 318). His figures for northern Britain (i.e. Scotland) were 72/5,554, a mortality of 1/77 (*ibid.*, pp. 338-9).

A detailed summary by the French physician Charles de la Condamine indicated the sort of variability in the results that were being obtained in the 1750s. His survey gives the following figures: 1/186 at the Foundlings Hospital, 1/370 at Winchester, 1/300 at Rye, 4/442 at Salisbury, 3/309 at Blandford, and 0/827 obtained by Ranby (La Condamine, 1755, pp. 18-19). If Ranby's results are included the overall mortality is 1/243, if they are excluded the figure is 1/160. According to La Condamine the differences were 'imputed to various degrees of malignity . . . to the several methods of preparing and treating the patients; to the different degrees of skill and experience of the inoculators . . . but principally to the observance or neglect of the maxim, not to venture inoculation upon subjects ill-disposed, unhealthy, or suspected of having other disorders' (La Condamine, 1755, pp. 19-20). Ranby's results were up-dated to 1/1,200 and his method, described by La Condamine (*ibid.*, pp. 24-6), can be taken as typical of those used by a successful variolator just before the Suttonian era. The patient was prepared by a few days' diet and medication. The material used was from a ripe pustule, taken from a healthy child and inserted into a slight incision. The patient was confined to his room during the eruption and attention was again paid to the diet.

The 1760s saw the rise of Daniel Sutton. Although claiming to be the originator of the Suttonian system he based his methods on those learned from his father Robert. Sutton was criticized for keeping his methods secret and, in fact, did not publish his own detailed account until 1796. Although he did keep the details of his methods and in particular his medicines secret, his results were widely publicized in the local newspapers and also by his associate the Rev. Robert Houlton who preached sermons in favour of variolation. An account of an unnamed system was published by Sir George Baker (1766) which Woodville identified as Sutton's system. Although Woodville considered that Houlton's sermons and pamphlets tended to exaggerate Sutton's success, he believed that Sutton's practice heralded a new era (Woodville, 1796, pp. 343–63).

Sutton shortened the preparatory period to two weeks, and advocated fresh air, exercise, and medicines during the eruptive illness. Although earlier workers, such as Ranby, had used a superficial incision, Sutton appears to have taken caution even further. He inoculated the 'smallest perceivable quantity', inserted in a manner that was 'barely sufficient to draw blood', with an incision 'not deeper that one-sixteenth of an inch' (Sutton, 1796, pp. 77–9). Van Zwannenberg (1978) has discovered an eye-witness account of the variolation of a young boy.

> The doctor [Sutton] thrust a lancet in one of them [the pustules providing the inoculum] which he immediately applied to the arm of Bamber and put so small a part of the point under the skin that he was not sensible of the points touching him. Then he put on his cloathes without plaister, rag or any covering whatever.

Sutton quickly made his fortune. His charge for inpatients was from £3.15 to £7.35, although the very well-to-do were charged £20. The poor were occasionally inoculated at no charge. It was estimated that Sutton earned 2,000 guineas in his first year and 6,000 in the second. Sutton's results were apparently so well-known by 1796 that he gave no detailed results on mortality in his account. According to Baker (1766, p. 22) a crude estimate was 6/17,000, i.e. 1/2,800. It has been claimed that Sutton and his immediate colleagues variolated 40,000 with only 5 deaths (van Zwannenberg, 1978). Another famous variolator who achieved remarkably low mortality rates was Thomas Dimsdale, whose method was based on that of Sutton although he placed more emphasis on exercise than medicine. Although we do not know how many he variolated he did say that only one patient died (Dimsdale, 1769, p. 1). He was so successful and respected that he was invited to Russia to variolate the Empress.

Although people such as Sutton, Dimsdale, and Ranby achieved remarkably low mortality rates there seems no reason to regard them as being representative. Even such a careful worker as John Haygarth obtained mortalities of 1/208 (Haygarth, 1785, pp. 197–8). There were also occasional disasters such as that at Blandford in 1766, when, of 384 variolated, 'a great number were in danger from the confluent smallpox and thirteen died' (Baker, 1766, pp. 57–8), a mortality rate of 1/30. George Pearson in his first monograph on vaccination listed data on the mortality from variolation at the end of the eighteenth century; William Heberden variolated 800 without any deaths and Woodville's figures for the first six months of 1798 were one death out of 1,700 variolations (Pearson, 1798, p. 67). Despite the results of Sutton, Dimsdale, Woodville, etc., some authoritative estimates for the overall mortality at the end of the eighteenth century are as high as 1/200, only three to four times less than at the introduction of variolation. Haygarth's actual figure was 1/208, and Pearson (1798, p. 67), Moore (1815, p. 302), and Robert Willan, the great dermatologist (Willan, 1806, p. 23), all gave 1/200 as their general estimate.

So there is no evidence from the data on mortality that smallpox virus was becoming *consistently* attenuated during variolation. Initially it had a mortality of 1/50–1/70 and by the end of the eighteenth century authoritative estimates gave a figure of about 1/200. There was considerable variation in the results and those obtained by Sutton, for example, indicated some considerable degree of attenuation which might indicate the emergence of vaccinia-like variants. This will have to be borne in mind whilst we consider the other factors.

The second factor which distinguished vaccination from variolation was its lack of communicability. However, claims that variolation did or did not transmit the disease have to be assessed in the light of what is now known about the communicability of natural smallpox. It is often said that smallpox is the most contagious of infectious diseases. This is not so; it is much less communicable than, for example, measles, influenza, or chickenpox. Smallpox is acquired naturally by inhaling virus shed by a patient with the disease. The infecting virus is commonly derived from the lesions in the mouth and less commonly from the virus in the skin vesicles. The scabs and crusts, although they contain much virus, are not an important source of infection as the virus needs to be released into the air in order to infect (Dixon, 1962, pp. 299–301). The possibility of airborne spread, other than to an immediately adjacent person, has always been a source of controversy and has been proved in very few cases (Werhle *et al.*, 1970); in most instances distant spread is thought to have been caused by a missed case or contaminated articles such as bedding.

Detailed investigation of both epidemic and endemic smallpox shows that the index case usually spreads infection to only very close contacts. Dixon (1962, pp. 408–48) gave a number of examples of the development of epidemics, and Henderson (1976b) estimated that one person generally infects only two to five other people. During an outbreak in London, in 1957, there were four undetected cases circulating in Greater London and each one only gave rise to one other case (Downie, 1970). Investigations on smallpox in family compounds in Nigeria have shown how slowly it spreads (Foege *et al.*, 1975). In one compound it took 53 days for all the four susceptible contacts to become infected; in another, 51 days to infect five susceptible contacts.

John Haygarth was greatly interested in the communicability of smallpox and concluded that infection was spread by contact or via infected articles or by the air, but only to close contacts. His 'Rules for Preventing the Smallpox' published in 1785 are still worth quoting in full (Haygarth, 1785, pp. 118–20).

I. Suffer no person, who has not had the smallpox to come into the infectious house. No visitor, who has any communication with persons liable to the distemper, should touch or sit down on anything infectious.

II. No patient, after the pocks have appeared, must be suffered to go into the street, or other frequented place. Fresh air must be constantly admitted by doors and windows into the sick chamber.

III. The utmost attention to cleanliness is absolutely necessary during and after the distemper, no person, clothes, food, furniture, dog, cat, money, medicine, or any other thing that is known or suspected to be bedaubed with matter, spittle, or other infectious discharges of the patient, should go or be carried out of the house till they be washed; and till they be sufficiently exposed to the fresh air. No foul linen, nor anything else that can retain the poison, should be folded up or put into drawers, boxes or be otherwise shut up from the air, but must be immediately thrown into water and kept there till washed. No attendant should touch what is to go into another family, till their hands are washed. When a patient dies of the smallpox, particular care should be taken that nothing infectious be taken out of the house so as to do mischief.

IV. The patient must not be allowed to approach any person liable to the disease, till every scab has dropt off; till all clothes, furniture, food, and all other things touched by the patient during the distemper, till the floor of the sick chamber, and till the hair, face and hands have been carefully washed. After everything has been made perfectly clean, the doors, windows, drawers, boxes, and all other places that can retain infectious air should be kept open, till it be cleared out of the house.

That variolation could transmit smallpox to others was demonstrated as early as 1721. Soon after the Newgate

Prison experiment Charles Maitland inoculated Mary Batt. She developed about fifteen pustules and recovered, but Maitland was greatly surprised to find that she infected six of the family's domestic servants. As there had been some doubt expressed about whether variolation really produced the smallpox in the inoculated person, the fact that the servants caught smallpox from Mary Batt was widely publicized. However, the leaflet printed to certify this, reproduced by Dixon (1962, p. 237), omitted to mention that one of the servants died.

From that time until variolation was made illegal in 1840 the fear that it might transmit smallpox to susceptible contacts was one of the main problems which prevented its unrestricted use. As natural smallpox is not very communicable, and inoculated smallpox might be expected to be less so, the fear was possibly misplaced but very real nevertheless.

In 1746 an Inoculation Hospital was founded in London and Woodville became its director in 1791. In 1800 he wrote of the '. . . spreading of the Smallpox from the inoculated, a circumstance which has greatly contributed to swell the bills of mortality for the metropolis, and of which the public has long justly complained' (Woodville, 1800, pp. 31–2). Sutton provided special inoculation houses for his fee-paying patients and restricted them to the grounds until they recovered. However, he was less careful with poor patients who were sent home. In 1765 he was put on trial at Chelmsford Assizes charged with spreading smallpox. He was acquitted because he convinced the jury that his patients had so few lesions that they could not have spread smallpox. The relationship between the severity of infection and communicability will be discussed later.

Thomas Dimsdale was probably even more famous than Daniel Sutton. Due to the success of his practice he was selected to visit Russia in 1768 to variolate the Empress Catherine and the Grand Duke Paul. The visit was a success, Dimsdale was created a Baron of the Empire and given £10,000 and an annuity of £500. For their equivalent value in 1979 these sums should be multiplied by about ten. He published his own account of his experiences in 1781 but a more accessible and readable account is given by Bishop (1932).

Dimsdale was a careful practitioner and in his writings repeatedly stressed the importance of preventing the spread of smallpox by variolated patients. Although no names are mentioned he possibly had Sutton in mind when he expressed surprise that some variolators allowed their patients 'to go abroad and follow their usual vocations' (Dimsdale, 1769, pp. 6–7).

The principal method adopted to prevent the spread of smallpox by variolation was by conducting what was usually known as a 'General Inoculation'. The method was outlined by Dimsdale as an example of how variolation could be introduced into Russia (1781, pp. 99–105). On a small scale he advocated the use of a separate house so that infection would not be transmitted to others. However, the aim of a general inoculation was to variolate large numbers at the same time, preferably by doing a whole village in one day. In this way everyone would be infected at the same time and there would be no susceptibles to whom infection could be spread. Those who were considered unsuitable for variolation were usually sent to an adjoining village or otherwise isolated.

Dimsdale's insistence on the importance of preventing the spread of smallpox caused by variolation led him into a lively pamphlet war. John Coakley Lettsom, the famous Quaker physician, and his friends were concerned that the poor were not being given the benefits of variolation, and they proposed a scheme for the free variolation of the poor of London in their own homes. Dimsdale opposed this on the grounds that it would do more harm than good by spreading the infection (Dimsdale, 1779). In all probability they were both right. Smallpox was endemic in London and most of the adult population would have already had it. It is doubtful whether any smallpox spread by variolation would have contributed significantly to the overall level of smallpox. However, in smaller towns and rural areas which were visited by smallpox only occasionally, variolation of isolated groups, or of whole villages, would be safer. However, the opposing views were based on belief rather than evidence that variolation did or did not spread smallpox, and such evidence as there was has to be interpreted in the light of modern evidence that natural smallpox is not very communicable.

Haygarth, whose rules for managing natural smallpox have already been quoted, advocated that they should also be used for controlling variolation, and proposed that a scheme of penalties and rewards be used to help enforce the rules (Haygarth, 1785, pp. 120–1; 1793, pp. 130–1). He reviewed evidence on the communicability of inoculated smallpox and his general conclusion was that it was transmitted only to close contacts. For instance, he published a letter sent to him from Geneva which reported that 'children so inoculated have gone freely into the streets, walks and other public places, before, during, and after the eruption, we have never observed that they were sources of contagion' (Haygarth, 1793, pp. 474–5). Haygarth thought that this was reasonable provided that the variolated patients did not come into contact with susceptible people. He argued that it was the fear of natural smallpox which kept susceptible people away from variolated people, 'for it is generally allowed that an inoculated patient, by a close approach, will communicate the casual infection' (*ibid.*, p. 493). Some of Haygarth's observations which demonstrated that variolation controlled smallpox rather than spread it have been recently misinterpreted. Razzell believes that such results 'can only be explained by assuming that inoculated cases were rarely a source of contagion' (Razzell, 1977b, p. 30). This is true, but the reason why they did not transmit infection was not just because of the low communicability but also because Haygarth took 'the most solicitous care . . . to prevent their communicating it to others' (Haygarth, 1793, pp. 187–8).

However, the main problem we are faced with is not whether variolation transmitted smallpox or even to what extent, but whether there is any evidence that it was becoming less communicable during the 70 years before vaccination was introduced. In view of the low communicability of natural smallpox and the conflicting views on inoculated smallpox it is not possible to reach a decision.

The third factor to consider is whether smallpox virus had been attenuated by variolation to the extent that it produced a single lesion at the point of insertion – a characteristic feature of vaccination. This problem is inseparably connected with that of communicability. In the years immediately following the introduction of variolation there was a belief that it was ineffective unless a full crop of pustules developed, and part of the criticism levelled at some of the improved methods was based on the belief that a single pustule would not confer immunity.

Sutton and other inoculators apparently managed to produce a single pustule at the site of inoculation in the majority of patients. However, it is not clear how closely their patients were examined. Smallpox consultants nowadays recommend the very close examination of a stripped patient in a good light so that the few small lesions of a mild case should not be missed. In many instances the variolators still referred repeatedly to the eruption in a very matter-of-fact way. Dimsdale for example referred to the eruption as 'the most interesting period of the distemper' (Dimsdale, 1769, p. 35). Sutton, writing with hindsight in 1796, said that by day nine 'we may about this time expect the eruption to make its appearance' (Sutton, 1796, p. 129), and gave instructions for the management of those 'uncomfortably burthened with pustules' (ibid., pp. 135–6).

We have seen that Sutton convinced the Chelmsford jury that his patients could not have spread smallpox because their eruptions were so sparse, and Haygarth believed that fewer lesions meant reduced communicability (Haygarth, 1793, pp. 486–7). Dimsdale, on the other hand, always took care to prevent those with very few pustules from mixing with the public (Dimsdale, 1769. p. 37).

Again we have to take account of up-to-date information on natural smallpox. Although strains of smallpox (variola major) from India were on the whole more virulent than those from South America (variola minor), the response in individual patients varied considerably. Consequently in an outbreak started by a single introduction of variola major, i.e. started by a single virus strain, there would be some very serious infections resulting in death and some very mild cases with very few lesions even in those who had never been vaccinated. Thus the mildness of smallpox, particularly in terms of the number of lesions, is almost as dependant on the response of the individual patient as on the strain of virus.

Whilst it is reasonable to propose that a patient with many lesions would be very likely to transmit infection, it does not necessarily follow that a person with very few lesions would not be very infectious. The reason for this is that, as explained previously, modern authorities regard respiratory virus as being more important than skin lesions in transmitting infection, and there are many accounts of patients with very few skin lesions who started epidemics. Christie, for example, tells of a patient with one lesion only who started an epidemic in which deaths occurred (Christie, 1969, p. 207).

The early variolators placed great stress on the effect of diet, medicines, and exercise in achieving a favourable result. Woodville, for example, believed that the introduction of mercury led to favourable results (Woodville, 1796, pp. 341–2). However, as controlled trials were not used and improved insertion methods were introduced at the same time, it is impossible to assess the validity of such claims. Many of the medicines contained high concentrations of mercury and/or antimony (Ruston, 1768), and Dixon has suggested that over-treatment might have done as much harm as good (1962, p. 245). In any event although treatment of the individual patient might have had some effect in modifying the severity of the infection produced, it could not have been expected to have any permanent effect on the virus.

Perhaps to modern investigators it is the virus that is the most interesting feature, because with to-day's live virus vaccines it is the careful selection and preservation of attenuated virus strains which is the important factor. For vaccinia-like strains to have emerged it would have been necessary for them to have been carefully conserved by arm-to-arm passage. However, there is no evidence that this happened; quite the reverse.

Woodville credits Frewen with the initial discovery that similar results were obtained with material from either natural or inoculated cases (Woodville, 1796, pp. 225–6). Ranby, one of the first to obtain low mortality rates used either method (La Condamine, pp. 24–6). Dimsdale took material from either the inoculation site or a natural pustule and obtained similar results. He did, however, emphasize that when he used a variolated donor he took virus from the inoculation site and not from a secondary pustule (Dimsdale, 1769. pp. 23–6). Haygarth who was interested in the whole concept of the control of infectious diseases, rather than narrowly concerned with variolation and who could perhaps be relied upon for an objective opinion, summed up the subject three years before the introduction of vaccination. 'Inoculating matter is taken indiscriminately from a good kind of inoculated or casual smallpox, and nobody has discovered or suspected any difference in their degree of virulence.' (Haygarth, 1793, p. 488). Such a practice which would randomly reintroduce 'wild' smallpox virus could not have been expected to lead to the emergence of stable vaccinial variants. In addition, whatever their evolutionary relationships, it is reasonable to regard variola minor as an attenuated type of variola major and there is no evidence that variola minor strains have become further attenuated this century so as to resemble vaccinia. It is perhaps also worth pointing out that there was no consistent reduction in the severity of natural smallpox during the eighteenth century. In fact in 1796, the year in which Jenner performed the first vaccination, the ratio of smallpox to other deaths in London was the highest of the century (Guy, 1882).

If vaccinia-like strains had emerged during the 1760s they would certainly have been recognized as such, particularly as so many people were looking for material with just the properties that vaccinia proved to have. It was not until the Jennerian era that such a virus was introduced. That it marked a complete break with previous practice is indicated by the way in which it was enthusiastically accepted by so many experienced variolators not only in England but also abroad. Limited attempts were made on the Continent to attenuate smallpox virus. These results which were also equivocal have been discussed by Genevieve Miller (1958). Post-Jennerian attempts to attenuate smallpox virus will be discussed in Chapter 11.

My conclusion, and not perhaps a very satisfactory one, is that smallpox virus could be sporadically modified by intradermal inoculation so as to produce a milder effect in the individual. Possibly, as Dixon suggested, the key factor was the growth of virus in the very superficial layers of the skin. The attenuation was probably due to the interaction between virus and host, and not due to any genetic change in the virus.

The overall impression left by an examination of the early literature is not so much the danger of variolation, though this was often stressed, but rather the variability and unreliability, and this impression is perhaps best summed up in the words of George Pearson;

> If an inoculator could, at his will, command on inoculation of the Smallpox, a slight local affection, a trifling eruptive fever, and a very small number of eruptions, there would be no temptation . . . to inoculate for the Cowpox (Pearson, 1798, p. 75).

One further aspect of early smallpox immunization needs to be mentioned – but only very briefly. This is whether

Jenner was the first to try inoculation of the cowpox. This is really a very minor point but some of Jenner's critics used this as part of their attempt to blacken his character. Originally Jenner made no claims to a discovery, but did so later, perhaps at the instigation of his friends, to counteract the claim of Pearson. However, it would have been surprising if he had been the first to test the milk-maid's folk-tale. Claims for priority were made by or on behalf of various people in England and Europe. Among these might be listed Fewster in 1765, Böse in 1769, Jesty in 1774, Nashe in 1781, and Platt and Jensen in 1791. Attempts were made by Jenner's critics, without any success, to show that he was aware of some of these earlier attempts. It is not uncommon now for the same observations to be reported quite independently by different workers, and it must have been even harder in the eighteenth century to be aware of what had been done.

Much has been made of the story of Benjamin Jesty, a Dorsetshire farmer who inoculated his wife and family with cowpox in 1774 (O'Malley, 1954). Jenner disbelieved the story for he thought it was being used to discredit him by Pearson. Jesty was brought to London in 1805 and fêted by the Original Vaccine Pock Institution which had been set up largely by Pearson. After his death Jesty was honoured by Crookshank who in 1889 used Jesty's portrait as the frontispiece of his *History and Pathology of Vaccination*.

However, despite these attempts to establish an earlier priority than Jenner's, the facts are simple. In all cases these claims did not come to light until after the publication of Jenner's monograph in 1798. If some of these early attempts were genuine they made no impact at all on medical opinion. If Jenner was not the actual 'discoverer' of vaccination, he was the one who first tested it and brought it to the attention of the public.

4

Edward Jenner

Just who was the man who was to be at the centre of one of the greatest ever medical controversies? Although most people will associate Jenner's name with smallpox vaccination, probably few will know that at the time he published his famous *Inquiry* he was 49 years old and had already made important contributions to science and medicine, including a unique observation of bird behaviour which although known by everyone, will be associated with Jenner's name by relatively few.

This is not intended to be a biography. However, as some of Jenner's critics made attacks on his other scientific work and on his character as a basis for their attacks on vaccination, his early career will need to be considered. Perhaps the most eminent of his later critics was Charles Creighton who, in his *Jenner and Vaccination* (1889), explained 'that the task which I set before me when I began this book was to explain to myself how the medical profession in various countries had come to fall under the enchantment of a dillusion'. As the Jenner centenary approached, Creighton's work was used as the basis of other attacks on Jenner. Almost all biographical information about Jenner comes from John Baron's two-volume *Life of Dr. Jenner* (1838). Baron was Jenner's friend and was given access to all his papers. His attempt to present Jenner as a man of genius has been correctly described as pathetic by Dixon, who suggested that Baron convinced Jenner, in his later years, of events which never really happened. It is against this view of Jenner the genius that Creighton's view of Jenner the rogue has to be balanced;

obviously the truth lies somewhere between the two. The biographies of Jenner which have been written this century, such as Drewitt's *Life of Edward Jenner* (1931) and especially Dorothy Fisk's *Dr. Jenner of Berkeley* (1959), are readable accounts with much personal detail, but tend not to go too thoroughly into scientific controversy. Dixon (1962), and Greenwood (1935, pp. 245–73) have brief but objective surveys, and the Jenner Centenary Issue of the *British Medical Journal* (1896) is very useful. For detailed information on Jenner's writings William Le Fanu's *Bio-bibliography of Edward Jenner* (1951) is invaluable.

Jenner was born on 17 May 1749, the third son of the Rev. Stephen Jenner of Berkeley, Gloucestershire; the patronage of the influential Berkeley family was to be of use to Jenner in later years. He attended local schools and showed interest in natural history, making collections of fossils and birds' nests. At thirteen he was apprenticed to Daniel Ludlow a surgeon-apothecary of Sodbury near Bristol, with whom he trained for about six years. He must have shown promise for he then became a student at St George's Hospital, London. Here he met the man who had the greatest influence on him – John Hunter.

Hunter was one of the giants of the age. An unsophisticated Scot, he had come to London in 1750 as a dissecting-room assistant to his brother William, who was already a well-known teacher and surgeon. John showed skill and aptitude and became a student at St Bartholomew's Hospital, London, and eventually became accepted as a teacher and surgeon himself. After four years' service as an Army surgeon he returned to London in 1763, entered private practice and set up a school of anatomy and surgery. He was elected FRS in 1767 and the following year appointed surgeon to St George's Hospital, London. He quarrelled with his brother William in 1780, claiming that the latter, who by then was being eclipsed by John, had given him insufficient credit for his help in the studies on the structure of the human placenta. Hunter is rightly regarded as one of the greatest surgeons and anatomists, but this tends to underestimate his more general contributions to comparative zoology, both anatomical and physiological.

In 1770 Jenner became one of Hunter's private house-students, along with Everard Home and Henry Cline, both of whom were to become Presidents of the Royal College of Surgeons. They attended classes and ward rounds at St George's and also Hunter's private classes. They also worked in Hunter's dissecting room helping him to perfect techniques for the preservation and display of specimens. Evidently Jenner showed some talent for this and when in 1771 Captain Cook arrived home from his first South Seas voyage with many specimens collected by Sir Joseph Banks, Hunter recommended that Jenner should arrange them. This job must have been done well for it was suggested that Jenner should accompany Banks as one of the naturalists to be taken on Cook's second voyage, but in the event neither Banks nor Jenner went. Nevertheless Jenner had made an influential contact in Banks, who was to be President of the Royal Society from 1778 until his death in 1820. Jenner returned to general practice in Berkeley in 1772. In 1775 Hunter offered Jenner a partnership in a scheme 'to teach natural history, in which will be included anatomy, both human and comparative'. Critics have pointed out that Hunter had already made the same offer to Daniel Ludlow's son who had declined it. However, that Hunter should have thought of Jenner at all is testimony to his skill. Hunter was obviously fond of and impressed by Jenner, and they exchanged letters until Hunter's death in 1793. Unfortunately none of Jenner's letters to him survive, but many of Hunter's letters do and are printed in Baron's biography. Those possessed by the Royal College of Surgeons have recently been published, many in facsimile, in an attractive pamphlet (*Letters*, 1976). In them Hunter bombards Jenner with requests for information and specimens and with suggestions for experiments. The impression gained is one of exciting haste:

Have you any caves where Batts go at night? . . . Have
you got the bones yet of a large Porpass I wish you had . . . I
have rec'd my Hedge Hogs . . . run the thermometer into
the anus and observe the heat; then open the belly by a
small hole and pass the thermometer down towards the
pelvis . . . Are hedgehogs in great plenty? I should like to
have a few . . . Have you any queer fish? . . . Send me all the
Fossels you find . . . Cannot you get me a large Porpass for
either Love or Money?

Many of Jenner's relatively incidental observations on
whales and hedgehogs were incorporated in Hunter's own
scientific papers.

Jenner's first independent publication was an account of a
new method for preparing Emetic Tartar, which he had
published anonymously in 1783. He also sent a copy to
Hunter under his own name and it was eventually published
again in 1793 (Jenner, 1793). Emetic tartar (antimony
potassium tartrate) was one of the many preparations of no
certain value used in an age when enforced vomiting and
bleeding were common procedures. Jenner's method
involved recrystallization of the salt to get a higher degree of
purity so that the dosage could be more exact. His product
was soluble in both water and wine. Emetic tartar is still
listed in Martindale's *Extra Pharmacopoeia* (1977) for use in
schistisomiasis and, dissolved in 'sherry-type' wine, as an
emetic, although the more soluble and less toxic sodium salt is
preferred. In an earlier generation it was recommended as a
general depressant, for acute eczema, fevers, and particularly
for catarrh and bronchitis (Ringer & Sainsbury, 1897).

Hunter was evidently pleased with his friend's product: 'I
also received your little publication with the Tart. Emet . . . I
approve of it much and will do all in my power to promote the
sale' and later 'The Physicians that I have given it to, speak
well of it as a more certain medicine than the other.'

Jenner also made fundamental observations on angina
pectoris in what were for him distressing circumstances.

Heberden in 1768 had described angina pectoris as a clinical entity, and Jenner had assisted Hunter when in 1772 he did the first autopsy on a case. Unfortunately the coronary arteries were not examined. From 1785 onward Hunter became increasingly ill and Jenner recognized in him the signs of angina pectoris. By this time he had himself performed autopsies on two cases and had recognized that thickening of the coronary arteries was a characteristic feature. He wrote to Heberden to tell him of his fears that Hunter had the disease, saying that he dared not tell Hunter – 'I am fearful that if Mr H. should admit this, that it may deprive him of the hopes of recovery'. After Hunter's death in 1793, his brother-in-law, Everard Home, wrote to Jenner describing the autopsy findings. 'It is singular that the circumstances you mentioned to me, and were always afraid to touch upon with Mr Hunter, should have been a particular part of his own complaint, as the coronary arteries were considerably ossified.'

In 1799 Caleb Parry of Bath published his famous *Inquiry into the symptoms and causes of the syncope anginosa, commonly called angina pectoris*. In it Parry generously credited Jenner with the suggestion that angina pectoris was caused by 'some morbid change in the structure of the heart, which change was probably ossification', and included in his book a letter from Jenner describing his experiences. Although Jenner emphasized the structural changes in the coronary arteries rather than the important functional changes recognized by Parry, he deserves credit for being the first to notice the structural changes and for being the first to associate them with clinical angina.

This brief account of angina, from 1768 to 1799, has taken us past 1789 in which year Jenner was elected to Fellowship of the Royal Society for some observations which many disbelieved and which still cast doubt on Jenner's scientific integrity. These were his *Observations on the Natural History of the Cuckoo*, published in the form of a letter to John Hunter (Jenner, 1788). It had been known for centuries that the cuckoo laid its eggs in the nest of another bird and that the eggs and young of the other bird were destroyed. However, it was not known how this was accomplished. Some thought that the parent ate her own young or ejected them from the nest; or that the young cuckoo used its superior strength to kill them, or that the other nestlings simply starved in the unequal competition for food.

Jenner had been studying cuckoos for many years, perhaps at Hunter's instigation, for this subject is mentioned in the earliest surviving letter from Hunter to Jenner, and further letters contain Hunter's promptings. 'I want the cuckoo cleared up . . . I request the whole history of the cuckoo . . . you must pursue the cuckoo.' Finally Jenner completed his observations in the 1786 season and submitted a paper to the Royal Society through Hunter in February 1787, and this was formally accepted the following month. The paper contained details of dissections of cuckoos and speculations on reasons for the cuckoo's behaviour. One original and very acute observation was that cuckoo eggs, which tend to be the same size and colour as those of the foster-parent, can be recognized through their being heavier. However, in this manuscript, which is in the possession of the Royal Society (Jenner, 1787), he concluded that it was the foster-parent which ejected its own young from the nest. Obviously he could not have seen this. It is clear that he could not keep nests under observation all the time and, in fact, some observations were made for him by his young nephew Henry. So his observations were, in fact, speculation on what happened since his last visit to the nest. He concluded:

> From these experiments, and supposing from the feeble appearance of the young cuckoo just disengaged from the shell that it was utterly incapable of displacing either the egg or the young sparrows I was induced to believe that the old sparrows were the only agents in this seeming unnatural business.

Why he submitted his speculations when he could so easily

have made accurate observations we can only guess. Perhaps he was exasperated by Hunter's increasingly insistent annual requests; perhaps his interest in cuckoos was waning. Perhaps he was becoming more interested in angina or cowpox or even in Catharine Kingscote whom he was to marry in 1788. In any event the first version presented unconfirmed speculation as fact and this episode is the strongest evidence used by those who were to accuse Jenner of being a lazy, unmethodical hoaxer. In any event Jenner's conscience must have pricked him because he continued his observations in the 1787 breeding season after submitting the paper. Perhaps he wanted to confirm his supposition so that he could anticipate publication of his paper with relief rather than anxiety. We can imagine his feelings when in June 1787 he saw what really happens – the newly-hatched cuckoo ejecting its fellow nestlings! He wrote to Banks asking that his manuscript be returned as he wanted to amend it. Then, following some frantic experiments with cuckoos' eggs in the last weeks of the season, the final version, incorporating his new and accurate observations was resubmitted in December 1787. The revised version was formally accepted in March 1788 and published shortly after. Jenner was hoping that this paper, on top of his previous work and with the support of Hunter and Banks would secure his election to Fellowship of the Royal Society. However, there was to be some delay, for as Hunter wrote to him 'the paper had better be first printed and delivered, and let the people rest a little upon it, for he [Sir Joseph Banks] says there are many who can hardly believe it wholly'. What they could not believe was that a newly-hatched cuckoo had the strength to lift the other nestlings, sometimes larger than itself, out of the nest.

The little animal, with the assistance of its rump and wings, continued to get the bird upon its back, and making a lodgement for the burden by elevating its elbows, clambered backward with it up the side of the nest till it reached the top, where resting for a moment, it threw off its load with a jerk, and quite disengaged it from the nest (Jenner, 1788, p. 225).

Jenner confirmed the crucial observation by placing cuckoos' eggs in nests and noting the result. He also saw two cuckoos' eggs in the same nest and described the fascinating competition between the two newly-hatched birds which resulted in the weaker being ejected.

This contest was very remarkable. The combatants alternately appeared to have the advantage, as each carried the other several times nearly to the top of the nest, and then sunk down again, oppressed by the weight of its burden; till at length, after various efforts, the strongest prevailed (*ibid.*, p. 229).

Jenner also described the unique anatomical feature which enabled the young cuckoo to perform its task.

The singularity of its shape is well adapted to these purposes; for, different from other newly-hatched birds, its back from the *scapulae* downwards is very broad, with a considerable depression in the middle. This depression seems formed by nature for the design of giving a more secure lodgement to the egg of the Hedge-sparrow, or its young one, when the young cuckoo is employed in removing either of them from the nest. When it is about twelve days old, this cavity is quite filled up, and then the back assumes the shape of nestling birds in general (*ibid.*, p. 226).

Jenner's account was accepted by most ornithologists but rejected by others and was a source of some discussion until unequivocally confirmed by cinematography in 1921. One person who totally disbelieved it was Creighton. He preferred Jenner's original view 'based on observations and abundantly confirmed', and concluded 'Jenner's cuckoo paper contains a few credible and prosaic facts; but the greater part of it and all that part of it which is best remembered, is a tissue of inconsistencies and absurdities' (Creighton, 1889, pp. 16–17). That Jenner's observations were 'absurd' was echoed later by Sir Norman Moore in his entry on Jenner in the *Dictionary of National Biography*.

It is *just* possible that Jenner may have chosen to use the most unlikely but correct explanation without actually making the observation, but it is inconceivable that he should invent the correct anatomical explanation. So Jenner's account proved to be correct and must have been based on accurate observation. However, the observations and the circumstances in which they were made were used by critics to prepare the way for attacks on vaccination. It was to become almost traditional for critics of Jenner to disbelieve him when it suited them and to interpret any ambiguous circumstance to his disadvantage.

Jenner was also involved in other researches, for example, on manures, ophthalmia, bird migration, and particularly tuberculosis. These are described by Le Fanu (1951). In addition some of Jenner's notebooks have survived and three have been published (Crummer, 1929; Drewitt, 1931; Hellman, 1931). They make fascinating reading and give an insight into the wide range of Jenner's interests.

Jenner obtained the degree of MD from St Andrews, Scotland, in 1792. In the manner of the times he had only to be recommended for the degree by two reputable physicians, and his friends John Hickes and Caleb Parry acted for him. Now able to style himself physician and surgeon, MD, FRS, he gave up general practice and became a private consultant, receiving patients referred to him by others. Parry, Hickes, and Jenner together with Thomas Paytherus had started a small medical society in 1788 called the Gloucester Medical Society. Some records of this society, listing papers presented by Jenner have survived and have been published (*British Medical Journal*, 1896). Jenner referred to this society as the 'medico-convivial society' to distinguish it from another, the 'convivio-medical society' which he also attended. The names give an idea of the order of priorities of the two societies. He could play the violin, drew well, and fancied himself as a poet – examples of his work are reproduced in his biographies and notebooks. He kept a good table, was a good host, and was well regarded both professionally and socially by a wide range of colleagues and friends.

It has usually been said that he disliked city life and preferred the life of a quiet country doctor. This might have been true of him when he declined Hunter's offer of a partnership in 1775 but not in later years. Although it is known that he used to spend some time in Cheltenham the extent of this has only recently been revealed by Paul Saunders (1969). Once Jenner had his MD and a growing reputation as a consultant he first rented in 1795, and then purchased, a home in Cheltenham and was listed as a resident physician in the Cheltenham Directory from 1800 to 1820. He was a member of the Cheltenham Commissioners (equivalent to the town council) from 1806 to 1821. Cheltenham at this time was a fashionable spa, and it is thought that Jenner's consultant friends in London found it convenient to be able to recommend a reliable physician to their patients who visited the spa. He apparently fitted well into the social circle and was founder and first president of the Cheltenham Literary and Philosophical Association. Only with the death of his wife in 1815 did he start to spend more time in Berkeley again. He had originally gone to Cheltenham to convalesce after a severe bout of typhus, and he had a similar infection in 1811. He was never very strong and the death of his wife affected him deeply. He went into semi-retirement in 1820 although he again started the paper on bird migration he had first started along with his cuckoo paper. He died in January 1823, four months before his 74th birthday.

A number of critical comments have been made about Jenner as part of the campaign to denigrate either him personally or vaccination in general, and some of these criticisms need to be discussed here.

A number of writers including Creighton, Dixon,

Greenwood, and even Jenner's anonymous biographer in the centenary *British Medical Journal* (1896), suggest that he was clumsy. The only evidence I know of, which supports such a claim, is found in a letter from Hunter in which he wrote, 'You very modestly ask for a thermometer; I will send you one but take care that those damned clumsy fingers do not break it also'. This, to me, is a typical example of Hunter's heavy-handed humour to be placed alongside the letter in which he agreed to be godfather to Jenner's son. 'I wish you Joy. It never rains but it pours. Rather than the brat should not be a Christian I will stand godfather, for I should be unhappy if the poor little thing should go to the Devel . . . I hope you begin to look grave now you are a father.'

Against this we have ample evidence of Jenner's skill. His work on the Banks specimens, the invitation to go on the second voyage, Hunter's offer of a partnership. Hunter was an outstanding anatomist with a particular interest in the preservation and display of specimens. Friendship notwithstanding, Hunter would not have considered Jenner for these tasks if he had not had sufficient technical skill.

Another criticism made of Jenner is that he was greedy. This is in connection with the petition presented to Parliament in 1802 for official recognition of his introduction of vaccination. There are at least two outstanding examples of his lack of greed. One was his refusal to benefit financially from his tartar emetic despite Hunter's urging that he do so. 'Do you mean to take out a Patint? . . . I would desire you to burn your Book for you will have all the world making it.' The other example, of course, is the reason for the petition itself – that he did not keep vaccination a secret. We have seen how both Dimsdale and Sutton profited from variolation, and Benjamin Waterhouse, who introduced vaccination into America, charged his fellow practitioners for vaccine until they were able to break his monopoly. Apparently none of Jenner's friends actively opposed his claim and he received support from such people as the Duke of Clarence, the Prime Minister (Addington), Lord Shelbourne, Admiral Berkeley,

William Wilberforce, Spencer Perceval, and Coakley Lettsom; the Prime Minister also let it be known that the King was in favour. Benjamin Travers wrote, 'If you had undertaken the extinction of the smallpox yourself. . . I am confident you might have put £100,000 in your pocket, and the glory be as great and the benefit to the community the same.' Witnesses giving evidence suggested that he might have made £20,000 per year from vaccination, and pointed out that he was actually put to some expense dealing with all his correspondence. There was some opposition to a financial reward but at the time his critics were more concerned with his claims of discovery and the question of the effectiveness of vaccination. In any event Jenner was voted £10,000, and an amendment to award him £20,000 was lost by three votes. He was awarded another £20,000 in 1807 (these figures should be multiplied by about 20 to give today's equivalent values).

There is no doubt that Hunter had a considerable influence on Jenner and it is probably true that Jenner was not his intellectual equal, despite the attempts of Baron to make him appear so. However, there is no reason to believe that he was as totally dependent on Hunter as has been suggested. His emetic tartar was original, his observations on angina pectoris were obviously kept from Hunter, and probably much of his cuckoo work was original if Hunter's many complaints and requests for information are to be believed. Hunter was no respecter of fools and it is unlikely that he would have offered Jenner a partnership if he had not had some respect for his friend. Finally despite all the criticism levelled at them Jenner's observations on vaccination made after Hunter's death were largely very sound.

Jenner has been accused of being lazy, particularly with respect to the cuckoo investigation, and it was argued by Creighton that Jenner's scientific output before he started work on vaccination, did not amount to much. However, Creighton was writing in another age and it is possible that Jenner saw life differently. With his diverse interests and a job to do he probably thought he was well occupied, and the snippets from his notebooks certainly support this conclusion. Many of the epithets used by Creighton to describe Jenner are almost mutually exclusive. If, as Creighton maintained, Jenner's cuckoo story and his later vaccinia work was all a 'sly, crafty, impudent' attempt to deceive, which largely succeeded, he could hardly have been the 'lazy, unmethodical, loose-minded shuffler' Creighton also accused him of being. Attention has been focused on Creighton's assessment of Jenner because it was such a vindictively personal one, and because coming as it did from a man of acknowledged intellect it served as a rallying point for a number of minor anti-vaccinationists at the time that the commemoration of the centenary of the first vaccination was about to be celebrated. It should be noted, however, that Crookshank, usually linked with Creighton as an influential critic, restricted his attack to Jenner the vaccinator.

A fair assessment of Jenner the scientist is that he was an acute observer, methodical in the manner of the times. Perhaps more of a theorist than an experimenter, he nevertheless had considerable technical skill. Although by no means a genius he was capable of pursuing original ideas in diverse fields. The one question mark against him must be his deliberate attempt to publish speculations on the cuckoo when accurate observations could have been made.

It is unfortunate that some have attacked Jenner the man as well as Jenner the scientist. To some he was too stubborn, to others he changed his ground. However, it is perhaps one of the engaging, if irritating, characteristics of the elderly, particularly when famous, that they possess both these characteristics and display which ever one suits. It is also said that he had an unpleasant personality and was difficult to get on with. However, fame, deserved or otherwise, does not neglect the boorish, and one can think of Nobel Prize winners who have been criticized for having these characteristics. In Jenner's case his critics point to his disagreement with George Pearson, arguments concerning the administration of the National Vaccine Establishment, petulant letters concerning friends who he thought were not supporting him, and more offensive letters about his opponents.

However, the fact that Jenner wrote in his private correspondence that a critic was 'a snarling fellow' has no relevance to the debate on whether the claims in Jenner's *Inquiry* or the criticisms of it were the most justified. Obviously where vaccination was concerned there was another side to Jenner. However, it probably amounts to little more than natural jealousy. After all, vaccination had completely changed his life at the age of forty-nine. It is evident that Pearson was attempting to attract credit which Jenner thought was unjustified, and it would have taken someone with the equanimity of a saint, which Jenner was not, to stand back and let Pearson take the credit.

Having set the scene we can now see what all the controversy was about.

5

Jenner's *Inquiry*

Jenner's first vaccination was performed on James Phipps on 14 May 1796. However, it is not clear how long his mind had been occupied with the problem. In his *Origin of the Vaccine Inoculation,* published in 1801, he mentioned that his inquiries had started 'upwards of twenty-five years ago' which would mean during the years after his stay in London with Hunter. According to Baron and Simon, Jenner's attention was drawn to the problem earlier whilst he was serving his apprenticeship with Ludlow. It is quite probable that he was told by a country girl that she considered herself secure from smallpox because she had already had cowpox, but it is unlikely that it was always at the front of his mind. Simon almost certainly exaggerated when he wrote that Jenner thought, and watched, and experimented on the subject for thirty years. However, there is some evidence that he was collecting information in those early years which was to be used in the *Inquiry*.* For example, he recorded that he was unsuccessful in his attempt to variolate Mrs H. in 1778 (*Inquiry,* Case V, pp. 14–15) and it is probable that in his attempts to ascertain the reason for this that she told him that she had cowpox many years before. He also mentioned that he had treated Hester Walkley when she had cowpox in 1782 (*Inquiry,* Case XII, p. 26).

By 1780 Jenner's ideas had crystallized sufficiently for him to discuss them with his friend Gardner and by 1788 he was

* *An Inquiry into the Causes and Effects of the Variolae Vaccinae,* Jenner, 1798. In this and later chapters references to this work will be introduced by the short title, *Inquiry,* with Case numbers and page references as indicated.

sufficiently confident to have an illustration of human cowpox made which he showed to his friends in London. These included Everard Home, Henry Cline, and Richard Worthington. Worthington told Haygarth who was very interested and expressed the hope that the matter would be investigated thoroughly (Crookshank, 1889, I, pp. 131–2). Although there is no direct evidence that Jenner discussed his ideas about cowpox with John Hunter, or when such discussions might have taken place, George Pearson mentioned that he had first heard of Jenner's ideas from Hunter in 1788 or 1789.

As an experienced practitioner Jenner would have been familiar with both natural and inoculated smallpox, and in 1789 he helped his colleague John Hickes in a small project which attracted the attention of the Gloucester Medical Society (*British Medical Journal*, 1896, p. 1297). Apparently a mild eruptive fever had appeared in Gloucestershire which the local people referred to as swinepox, pigpox, or cowpox. There was some doubt in the minds of the medical men as to whether the disease was a mild form of smallpox or something else. The nurse who was attending Jenner's son Edward had the disease, and from her Jenner and Hickes inoculated young Edward and also two servants who had never had smallpox or chickenpox. The result was similar to inoculated smallpox but perhaps a bit more severe. About a month later the three were variolated but this had no effect, so it appears that the swinepox was a variety of smallpox. It evidently interested the members of the Society and they drew up proposals to collect further information on the subject. Jenner also started to draft out a paper on it which was later to be incorporated into the *Inquiry* (*Inquiry*, pp. 54–5). However, we hear nothing more of it at the time. Possibly by now Jenner really was interested in cowpox and collecting the case histories which he was to use to support his hypothesis.

Before dealing with the published *Inquiry* a little should be said about the earlier, unpublished version. This was one of the principal stimuli which led Crookshank to investigate the history of vaccination and was discussed by him in detail (Crookshank, 1889, 1, pp. 250–65). In 1888 Crookshank discovered the manuscript of a paper which Jenner had sent to the Royal Society and which was obviously an alternative version of the cowpox story which had been written in 1796. It had been given, along with some other papers, to the library of the Royal College of Surgeons by Sir James Paget, and its importance had not been recognized. Crookshank published long extracts in his *History* and the whole of it was published in 1923, the centenary of Jenner's death (Jenner, 1923). This manuscript described the case histories of thirteen people who had resisted variolation or natural smallpox after having cowpox. It also described the vaccination of Phipps. Crookshank believed that alterations, in another hand, had been made to the paper. In particular he was impressed by the fact that on page 42 of the manuscript the word 'discovery' had been replaced by 'investigation', thus suggesting to Crookshank that some critic had pointed out to Jenner that no discovery had been made. This page has been reproduced and Crookshank's claim that the alterations were not made by Jenner was rejected (*British Medical Journal*, 1896, pp. 1257–9).

Crookshank also believed that this manuscript had been rejected by the Royal Society. However, he was probably incorrect for there is no evidence in the Society's comprehensive records that the manuscript was ever formally received. Jenner had sent the paper to Everard Home, who was on the Council of the Society, hoping that it would be acceptable for publication. Home showed it to Sir Joseph Banks, and to Lord Somerville, the President of the Board of Agriculture. They apparently thought that there was insufficient evidence to support such important claims, and suggested that it might spoil Jenner's reputation to publish it without further evidence. Jenner obtained further evidence in 1798 and, perhaps not wishing to risk another snub, published his findings at his own expense. His monograph appeared in June 1798 with the full title *An Inquiry into the Causes and Effects of the Variolae Vaccinae, a Disease Discovered in some of the Western Counties of England, particularly Gloucestershire, and known by the name of the Cowpox.*

Although the four books, written by Jenner between 1798 and 1801, represent the whole of his basic contribution to the subject of vaccination, it is probably better to consider the *Inquiry* on its own first. After all, this was all the earliest workers had available with which to assess Jenner's claims, and from a historical point of view later critics have taken the same approach. Jenner's later books appeared after George Pearson had published his own *Inquiry* and after the vaccines introduced by William Woodville had been described in the first of his pamphlets. Consequently Jenner's later publications are probably best regarded as being his contributions to the controversy with Woodville which will be discussed in detail in a later chapter.

Jenner made a number of claims in his *Inquiry*. These claims, and the evidence on which they were based were to be a source of controversy for many years, and the reception which the *Inquiry* received will be described in the next chapter. The *Inquiry* can, for convenience, be divided into four sections. The first, which may be regarded as an introduction, gives a brief account of cowpox (*Inquiry,* pp. 1–7). In the second section Jenner described instances in which 28 people who had suffered from cowpox at some time in the past had subsequently resisted either natural or inoculated smallpox. The 28 people were grouped into 15 'Cases' (*Inquiry,* pp. 9–30). Case XVI provided a link between the second and third sections because it was from this patient that the material used to perform the first vaccination was obtained. The third section comprised Jenner's practical experience of what was soon to be known as vaccination. One vaccination was done in 1796 and the remainder as a linked series in 1798 (pp. 32–44). The final section is a long rambling discussion which, in Jenner's own words, made 'some general observations on the subject and on some others which are interwoven with it'.

The most important claim was, of course, that 'the Cow-pox protects the human constitution from the infection of the Small-pox'. The circumstantial evidence on which this conclusion was based is to be found in Cases I to XII; of these, Case VI comprised three people, Case VII four, and Case XII eight. The actual vaccinations whicn confirmed his theory were described in Cases XVII and XIX to XXIII.

It is not known how many of the cases of cowpox Jenner actually saw himself. Some had occurred many years before and, although some dates were given, others have to be calculated from the time intervals mentioned. He could not have seen Cases III, IV, and VIII, nor probably Case V because they occurred before he started his apprenticeship with Ludlow. Cases I, II, IX, and X occurred between 1767 and 1782 in the Berkeley area and he could have attended them. Alternatively he could have been given first-hand information by colleagues. Jenner mentioned that he attended Case XVI and one of the patients in Case XII, and it is likely that he saw the seven individuals in Cases VI and VII because they occurred in the summer of 1796, the year of his first vaccination, when his interest must have been high.

Resistance to smallpox was determined by variolation or by exposure to natural smallpox or both. The tests would have been invalidated if any of the patients had already had smallpox before having cowpox. However, Jenner took the 'utmost care' to ensure that none of the people in his survey had previously had smallpox. The investigations were made in a rural area with a sparse population which was visited only occasionally by smallpox 'and where such an event as a person's having had the Small Pox is always faithfully recorded, no risk of inaccuracy in this particular can arise' (*Inquiry*, p. 10).

It is not clear how many of the variolations were done by Jenner. He certainly variolated the twelve people described in Cases I, III, V–VIII, and X, and mentioned that the eight

CASE XI.

WILLIAM STINCHCOMB was a fellow fervant with Nichols at Mr. Bromedge's Farm at the time the cattle had the Cow Pox, and he was unfortunately infected by them. His left hand was very feverely affected with feveral corroding ulcers, and a tumour of confiderable fize appeared in the axilla of that fide. His right hand had only one fmall fore upon it, and no fore difcovered itfelf in the correfponding axilla.

[25]

In the year 1792 Stinchcomb was inoculated with variolous matter, but no confequences enfued beyond a little inflammation in the arm for a few days. A large party were inoculated at the fame time, fome of whom had the difeafe in a more violent degree than is commonly feen from inoculation. He purpofely affociated with them, but could not receive the Small Pox.

During the fickening of fome of his companions, their fymptoms fo ftrongly recalled to his mind his own ftate when fickening with the Cow Pox, that he very pertinently remarked their ftriking fimilarity.

Figure 2 Jenner's account of the unsuccessful variolation of William Stinchcomb, Case xi of the *Inquiry*. (Liverpool Medical Institution).

people in Case XII were variolated by his nephew and assistant, Henry Jenner. All the others were variolated in the Berkeley area and could have been done by the Jenners or by close colleagues. All the cases except Case XVI were tested by variolation. Cases I, II, IV, and IX were also exposed to natural smallpox, and Cases X–XII also associated with people who had smallpox by variolation. The amount of detail given in the cases varied but on the whole was not extensive. Case XI, which describes the cowpox infection and subsequent variolation of William Stinchcomb, is reproduced in Figure 2.

Case XVI was Sarah Nelmes who became infected with cowpox in May 1796. Unfortunately she was not variolated but Jenner considered that 'the pustule was so expressive of the true character of the Cow-pox, as it commonly appears upon the hand' that he included an engraving of it in the *Inquiry* which is reproduced here (Figure 3). Jenner used

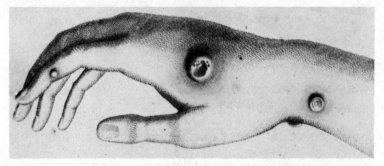

Figure 3 Accidental human cowpox, 1796. The lesions on the hand of Sarah Nelmes, Case XVI of Jenner's *Inquiry*. (Liverpool University).

material from Nelmes to vaccinate James Phipps, 'a healthy boy, about eight years old' (*Inquiry*, Case XVII, pp. 32–4). The results were 'much the same as when produced in a similar manner by variolous matter', although the area surrounding the lesion had 'more of an erysipelatous look than we commonly perceive when variolous matter has been made use of in the same manner'. Phipps complained of uneasiness in the axilla, and had some general discomfort from day seven to day nine but quickly recovered. In July he was variolated on both arms. 'The same appearances were observable on the arms as we commonly see when a patient has had variolous matter applied, after having either the Cow-pox or the Small-pox.' He was variolated again several months later, again without effect. Phipps became Jenner's most celebrated patient and was set up in a cottage in Berkeley which now houses a museum run by the Jenner Trust. Jenner variolated Phipps many times to demonstrate his immunity to smallpox. However, the continued resistance was likely to have been boosted by those variolations which could be regarded as a series of re-vaccinations, and as such gave no real indication as to the effectiveness of the original vaccination.

Jenner continued his experiments two years later in March 1798. The sequence of vaccinations is shown in Figure 4. Thomas Virgoe contracted cowpox, apparently from a horse

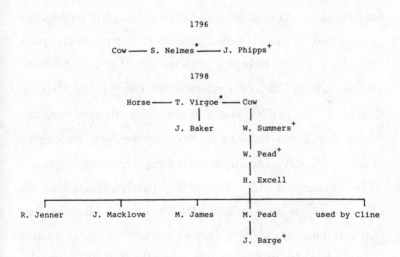

*Nelmes and Virgoe were infected accidentally

+These patients successfully resisted variolation

Figure 4 Chart showing the vaccinations done by Jenner in 1796 and 1798. Hannah Excell was the only person named of those who were vaccinated from Pead.

(see later) and from him material was used on 16 March to vaccinate John Baker, a five-year-old (*Inquiry*, Case XVIII, pp. 35–7), whose arm was illustrated in an engraving. Baker could not be variolated due to him 'having felt the effects of a contagious fever in a work-house'. In fact Baker died, as Jenner was later to admit. This episode, as will be described in the next chapter, was to be severely criticized.

William Summers (*Inquiry*, Case XIX, pp. 37–8) aged five-and-a-half was vaccinated at the same time as Baker, but with material from a cow which was infected in the same outbreak which involved Virgoe and the horses. Summers 'became

CASE XX.

FROM William Summers the difeafe was transfered to William Pead a boy of eight years old, who was inoculated March 28th.   On the 6th day he complained of pain in the axilla, and on the 7th was affected with the common fymptoms of a patient fickening with the Small-pox from inoculation, which did not terminate 'till the 3d day after the feizure.   So perfect was the fimilarity to the variolous fever that I was induced to examine the fkin, conceiving there might have been fome eruptions, but none appeared. The efflorefcent blufh around the part punctured in the boy's arm was fo truly characteriftic of that which appears on variolous inoculation, that I have given a reprefentation of it.   The drawing was made when the puftule was beginning to die away, and the areola retiring from the centre. (See Plate, No. 3.)

Figure 5 Jenner's account of the vaccination of William Pead, Case xx of the *Inquiry*. (Liverpool Medical Institution).

indisposed on the 6th day, vomited once, and felt the usual slight symptoms till the 8th day, when he appeared perfectly well'. Jenner noted that the lesion lacked the livid tint seen in Phipps. Virus from Summers was used on 28 March to vaccinate William Pead (*Inquiry*, Case XX, p. 38). The account is reproduced in Figure 5 and the engraving in Figure 6. As can be seen Jenner was struck by the similarity of the general symptoms to those of variolation, and by the similarity of the 'efflorescent blush' surrounding the lesion to that which accompanied variolation.

On 5 April the virus from William Pead was used to

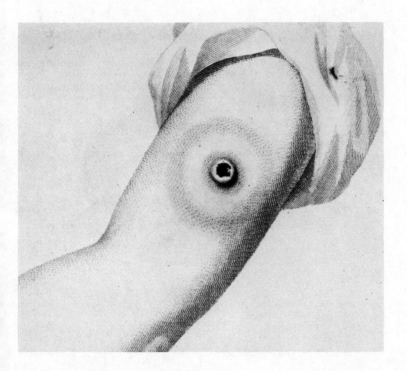

Figure 6 The engraving of the vaccination lesion on the arm of William Pead, Case XX of the *Inquiry*. (Liverpool University).

vaccinate 'several children and adults' (*Inquiry*, Case XXI, pp. 39–40). Three of these apparently had severe reactions with 'extensive erysipelatous inflammation' and in two of them this was controlled by the use of mercurial ointment. Only one patient was named, Hannah Excell, one of the patients without erysipelatous inflammation, who was vaccinated at three sites. According to Jenner her lesions 'so much resembled, on the 12th day, those appearing from the insertion of variolous matter, that an experienced Inoculator would scarcely have discovered a shade of difference at that period'. An engraving of Excell's lesions was included and is reproduced here (Figure 7). As will be discussed in the next

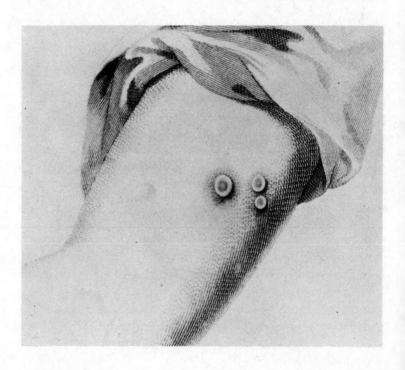

Figure 7 The engraving of the vaccination lesions on the arm of Hannah Excell, Case XXI of the *Inquiry*. Excell was vaccinated at three sites. (Liverpool University).

chapter these lesions are sufficiently different from those of inoculated smallpox to require specific comment.

Virus from Excell was used to vaccinate four children (*Inquiry*, Case XXII, pp. 40-2). One of them, Jenner's son Robert, did not respond. The other three did and Jenner, fearing that their arms might be as bad as the ones just mentioned, applied a mixture of quick-lime and soap to two of them for six hours. However, the arm of the third healed without any undue symptoms. Virus from this third patient, Mary Pead, was used to vaccinate the last in the series, J. Barge (*Inquiry*, Case XXIII, p. 42), who went through the disease 'with the usual slight symptoms'. Thus the vaccination of William Summers on 16 March was the start of a series of vaccinations in which the vaccine was passed through a series of four arm-to-arm transfers.

Unfortunately Jenner, perhaps deserving the accusation that he was lazy, did not think it necessary to test all the vaccinated patients by variolation. However, he did appreciate the importance of testing Summers and Barge who were the first and last in the serial series. Jenner himself variolated Summers but with no effect. Jenner's nephew Henry variolated Barge and also William Pead. Because the interpretation of these variolations was to be contested and as Henry Jenner gave a reasonably full account, it is worth quoting in full.

I have inoculated Pead and Barge, two of the boys whom you lately infected with the Cow-pox. On the 2d day the incisions were inflamed and there was a pale inflammatory stain around them. On the 3d these appearances were still increasing and their arms itched considerably. On the 4th day, the inflammation was evidently subsiding, and on the 6th it was scarcely perceptible. No symptoms of indisposition followed.

To convince myself that the variolous matter made use of was in a perfect state, I at the time inoculated a patient with some of it who had never gone through the Cow-pox, and it produced the Small-pox in the usual regular manner (*Inquiry*, p. 43).

Jenner also suggested that for cowpox to exert its protective effect it had to produce 'tumours in the axillae . . . and general indisposition' in addition to the local lesion. His evidence for this was one patient at the end of the *Inquiry* (*Inquiry*, p. 71) who had a local lesion only and who had subsequently had a mild attack of naturally-acquired small-pox.

So the evidence on which Jenner's principal claim was made comprised 25 cases of cowpox, 24 of whom were tested and found to resist variolation, and a number of people who were vaccinated, four of whom were resistant to variolation. We do not know exactly how many were vaccinated; it was nine plus the several adults and children of Case XXI.

One of the controversies into which Jenner was soon to be drawn was the length of the period of immunity to smallpox which vaccination conferred. In his own words Jenner pointed out that 'what renders the Cow-pox virus so extremely singular is, that the person who has been thus affected is for ever after secure from the infection of the Small-pox'. This was a rash claim. To support it Jenner selected in some of his cases people whose cowpox infection had occurred many years before they successfully resisted variolation. For example, for Joseph Merret (Case I) the interval was 25 years, for Sarah Portlock (Case II) it was 27 years, John Philips (Case III), 53 years, Mary Barge (Case IV), 30 years, and for Elizabeth Wynne (Case VIII), whose cowpox was mild, the interval was 38 years.

Another controversy which as we will see later will probably never be resolved, was Jenner's claim that 'the source of the infection [i.e. cowpox] is a peculiar morbid matter arising in the horse'. In the *Inquiry* (*Inquiry*, p. 2) Jenner very briefly described a disease of horses called the *grease*, 'an inflammation and swelling in the heel, from which issues matter possessing properties of a very peculiar kind'.

He went on to explain that the grease could be transferred accidentally to cows when men who had been tending sick horses then went to help with the milking. The infection in cows was called *cowpox*, and people who had caught this infection formed the cases discussed above. Jenner also listed three men (*Inquiry*, Cases XIII–XV, pp. 27–30) who had become infected directly from sick horses. However, their responses to variolation were not consistent. The virus which was used in the main series of vaccinations was said to have originated from a sick horse. As mentioned above John Baker (Case XVIII) was inoculated with virus from lesions on the hand of Thomas Virgoe who had been tending a mare with sore heels. One of Virgoe's colleagues, Haynes, who had also been infected from the mare, apparently transferred the infection to the cows he was helping to milk and the virus from one of these cows was used to initiate the series of vaccinations described earlier.

The evidence that grease was the real origin of cowpox was circumstantial, but the idea seemed to catch Jenner's imagination although he admitted that he had 'not been able to prove it from actual experiments'. However, as mentioned above, the variolation of the three men who had been accidentally infected with grease directly from horses gave variable results whereas those infected from cows consistently resisted variolation. Of the three infected directly one, Thomas Pearce (*Inquiry*, Case XIII, pp. 27–8) successfully resisted variolation after six years. The second, James Cole (*Inquiry*, Case XIV, p. 28) became infected at the same time as Pearce, but variolation after four years produced a slight eruption which Jenner interpreted as indicating only partial resistance. The third person, Abraham Riddiford (*Inquiry*, Case XV, pp. 29–30) in an unrelated episode contracted a severe infection from a horse, and had a mild attack of natural smallpox twenty years later. These results may well just indicate the almost inevitable variability of uncontrolled biological experiments. However, Jenner concluded that 'the active quality of the virus from the horses' heels is greatly increased after it has acted on the nipples of the cow'. In other words although grease was the origin of cowpox, vaccine could only be relied upon which had come from the cow.

Another controversial claim was that 'it is singular to observe that the Cow-pox virus, although it renders the constitution unsusceptible of the variolous, should nevertheless, leave it unchanged with respect to its own action'. The evidence of this claim was that William Smith (*Inquiry*, Case IX, pp. 21–2) apparently had cowpox in 1780, 1791, and 1794, but was variolated without effect in 1795. Other evidence was provided by Elizabeth Wynne (*Inquiry*, Case VIII, pp. 20–1; 51) who had cowpox in 1759, resisted variolation in 1797, and had a relatively severe attack of cowpox in 1798. A related observation which also caused some surprise was that people who had previously had smallpox were still susceptible to cowpox. In Cases VI and VII Jenner described five farmworkers who caught cowpox although they had all previously had natural smallpox. In addition Virgoe and Haynes who were infected from the horses had previously been variolated.

In all the observations and claims described so far Jenner assumed that the viruses which caused the grease, the cowpox in cows, and the single and repeated attacks of human cowpox were identical. This work was done long before viruses were discovered and also before the importance of working with purified preparations was appreciated. In addition epidemiological investigations were still in their infancy. We know now that there are other animal poxviruses, some of which are immunologically related to cowpox and smallpox yet biologically distinct. Consequently we would still accept most of Jenner's claims if the viruses involved were not identical but just immunologically related. The possibility that biologically different but immunologically related viruses were circulating in the eighteenth and nineteenth centuries will be discussed in Chapter 12. However, Jenner suspected that viruses, immunologically quite distinct from cowpox, might cause confusion and he emphasized the importance of using the correct material. This led him into another controversy. In the introductory pages of the *Inquiry* Jenner briefly described the course of cowpox in both man and cow. In the cow it produced irregular pustules with a pale-blue tint which became surrounded by erysipelatous inflammation. They frequently degenerated into 'phagedenic ulcers'. In human cases the lesions started as inflamed spots which resembled burns and then produced depressed bluish vesicles. There were some constitutional symptoms such as pains in the axillae 'shiverings with general lassitude and pains about the loins and limbs with vomiting . . . The head is painful and the patient is now and then affected with delirium.' The extent of these symptoms varied in different individuals and lasted from one to four days. The lesions healed slowly, and frequently became phagedenic as in the cow (*Inquiry*, pp. 3–7). In a footnote to page 7 Jenner described another infection which he said occurred in the cow spontaneously, i.e. no connection with horses was suspected. This infection was always free of the 'bluish or livid tint' which was so characteristic of cowpox, and did not confer resistance to smallpox. This infection was to become one of several kinds of 'spurious' cowpox, a term which was to be used repeatedly during the nineteenth century to explain away apparently unsuccessful or too severe vaccinations. This subject will be considered in detail in Chapter 10.

As an experienced variolator Jenner was aware of the need for a safe alternative to variolation. His opinion was 'that notwithstanding the happy effects of Inoculation . . . it not very infrequently produces deformity of the skin, and, sometimes, under the best management, proves fatal'. He discussed those features which appeared to make cowpox inoculation a safe alternative to variolation. Firstly, no fatalities had resulted from cowpox 'even when impressed in the most unfavourable manner'. Secondly, it did not cause a generalized pustular eruption. Thirdly, it did not 'seem possible for the contagious matter to produce the disease from effluvia, or by any other means than contact . . . so that a single individual in a family might at any time receive it without the risk of infecting the rest or of spreading a distemper that fills a country with terror' (*Inquiry*, pp. 66–8).

Finally, we may see what Jenner thought of the relationship between cowpox and smallpox. Obviously there must be some relationship because he had shown that cowpox conferred immunity to smallpox. He asked:

> May it not, then, be reasonably conjectured, that the source of the Small-pox is morbid matter of a peculiar kind, generated by a disease in the horse, and that accidental circumstances may have again and again arisen, still working new changes upon it, until it has acquired the contagious and malignant form under which we now commonly see it making its devastations amongst us? (*Inquiry*, pp. 53–5).

As will be explained later, the one feature of the *Inquiry* which triggered Creighton's flood of criticism was, to him, Jenner's unexplained and unjustified use of the term *variolae vaccinae*, i.e. smallpox of the cow. In the *Inquiry*, although Jenner stressed the advantages of cowpox inoculation over variolation, he also emphasized the similarities between the two whereas, as will be explained later, others were to stress the differences. This is particularly true of the precise appearance of the lesion.

As mentioned earlier Jenner was probably not the first to inoculate cowpox and test its protective effect, and so in that sense he was not a discoverer. He was, however, the first to publish an account of the phenomenon. Although the word 'discovered' was used in the title, no specific claims of discovery were made. In the dedication of the *Inquiry* to Caleb Parry (later editions were dedicated to the King), Jenner mentioned that 'it is remarkable that a disease of so peculiar a nature as the Cow Pox, which has appeared in this and some of the neighbouring counties for such a period of years, should so long have escaped particular attention'.

Perhaps the most important practical observation, apart from the basic demonstration that cowpox protected against smallpox, was that 'the matter in passing from one human subject to another, through five gradations lost none of its original properties'*. This method of arm-to-arm vaccination meant that fresh material did not have to be continuously obtained from the cow, and this was to be the method used to propagate vaccine until late in the nineteenth century.

In the final paragraph Jenner admitted that his investigations were incomplete and hoped that the combination of experiment and conjecture would 'present to persons well situated for such discussions, objects for a minute investigation. In the mean time I shall myself continue to prosecute this inquiry, encouraged by the hope of its becoming essentially beneficial to mankind' (*Inquiry*, pp. 74–5).

This then was Jenner's *Inquiry* which was to become such a source of controversy. Although much of the evidence was circumstantial, many of the points made were far more accurate than Jenner's critics realized. In particular his observations on true and spurious cowpox, as we shall see, were far in advance of the critical analyses made of them at the end of the nineteenth century. It is likely that these were the result of inspiration and acute observation on Jenner's part, rather than the careless work of a loose-minded unmethodical man, such as he was to be accused of being.

---

* In fact there were only four arm-to-arm transfers, although there were five transfers from the cow through to J. Barge (*see* Figure 4, p. 59).

6

Reactions to the *Inquiry*

The publication of the *Inquiry* did not come as a surprise. Pearson referred to it as 'long-expected', and the idea that cowpox might protect against smallpox was mentioned very briefly by Adams in 1795 and Woodville in 1796. It appears that they had been provided with information by Jenner's friend Henry Cline.

It would take a whole book to examine adequately the reactions to the claims made in the *Inquiry*. All that can be done here is to assess the earliest reactions by Jenner's contemporaries, and also the reactions of his most influential critics a century later, and to see how reasonable the claims and criticisms made of them appear in the light of present-day information.

When Jenner visited London to arrange for publication of the *Inquiry* he had brought vaccine with him but was unable to interest anyone sufficiently to try it. The first confirmation came almost by accident. He had left some vaccine with Cline who had a young patient with a diseased hip. Cline inoculated the vaccine in the hope that it might encourage a discharge from the hip. The vaccination took and the patient resisted subsequent variolation. The vaccine had been taken from Hannah Excell in April and had been successfully stored for about three months, dried in a quill (Baron, 1838, I, pp. 151–3).

Perhaps the first hint of trouble in store came in October 1798 with a letter from Dr John Ingenhousz. This episode was typical of the kind of hasty reaction by authoritative critics to which Jenner over-reacted, thus attracting further criticism to himself. Ingenhousz, who had been a pupil of Dimsdale, had a particular interest in smallpox and variolation and had introduced variolation into Austria. He had variolated the Empress Maria Theresa and was now physician to the Emperor. He was visiting the Marquess of Lansdowne in Wiltshire when the *Inquiry* appeared. Although he had no first-hand knowledge of cowpox he obtained hearsay evidence from local practitioners who advised him that in their experience it did not protect against smallpox. In the *Inquiry* (1798, pp. 56–8) Jenner had suggested that improper storage of the smallpox virus used by variolators had occasionally led to putrefaction so that the lesion produced would not confer immunity. Ingenhousz informed Jenner that 'by inquiring more minutely' he would 'find it erroneous', and Creighton was to refer to the idea as absurd. However, the possibility that early vaccines might have been contaminated with pyogenic bacteria is very high. Jenner tried to convince Ingenhousz that his results were genuine and that any smallpox must have followed spurious cowpox. The exchange of letters was published by Baron (1838, 1, 291–300).

Dr John Sims, a reputable London physician, published a letter early in 1799 in which he wrote of a man who had apparently had cowpox twice and 'being afterwards inoculated for the smallpox, had it in so great abundance that his life was for some time despaired of' (Sims, 1799). He afterwards conceded that the cowpox might have been spurious. A similar account was also reported by Mr Cooke, an apothecary from Gloucester. Cooke's patient was 'so ill with fever, and these boils, that she could not work for a week', but many years later had smallpox by inoculation (Cooke, 1799).

Probably the first published examination of Jenner's *Inquiry* appeared in November 1798. It was written by George Pearson who quickly collected information from a number of correspondents and published it as *An Inquiry Concerning the History of the Cowpox Principally with a View to Supercede and Extinguish the Smallpox*. Pearson, a physician and teacher at St George's Hospital, London, although a supporter of vaccination, was soon to be involved with Jenner in an argument over the administration of Vaccine Institutes and was later to challenge Jenner's Parliamentary Petition.

Many of his correspondents had some knowledge of cowpox although it was apparently unknown in Cheshire, Lancashire, Lincolnshire, Yorkshire and Durham. However, those of his correspondents who had heard of it recognized that it did confer immunity to smallpox (Pearson, 1798, pp. 7–13; 29–37). Pearson tried to find some cowpox himself but the only case he found had almost healed and attempts to inoculate eight volunteers failed. He did however find three men who were believed to have had cowpox but not smallpox. These were variolated by staff of the Smallpox Hospital using virus supplied by Woodville. The three test volunteers had no generalized lesions and the local lesion became inflamed with possibly a small vesicle in two and a little scab in the other. In each case the slight reaction 'seemed too rapid for that of the variolous infection when it produces the smallpox'. In other words the result was the typical accelerated take which denotes immunity. Two additional volunteers who had never had smallpox were variolated to provide a control. These had mild smallpox, one with twenty or thirty pustules and the other with about a dozen (Pearson, 1798, pp. 14–26).

There is no reason to suppose that at this stage anyone but Jenner and his closest colleagues had any vested interest in demonstrating the effectiveness of vaccination. Consequently these results of Pearson's must be seen as independent confirmation of Jenner's claim that those who had cowpox accidentally were resistant to smallpox.

However others throughout the nineteenth century were to assert that cowpox did not protect or at best that it exerted only a temporary non-specific effect. The basis of the criticism was the interpretation of the *variolous test* which was discussed at length by Creighton (1889, pp. 126–54). Creighton and those who were influenced by him such as the Dissentient Royal Commissioners saw a similarity between the effects of the 'improved' methods of variolation which were said to produce a very mild infection and protection against subsequent smallpox, and the effects of the variolation which was used to test the effectiveness of vaccination. In this latter instance the variolation was said to have produced a negligible result and indicated that the vaccine had produced immunity to it. I think, however, that Creighton over-emphasized these similarities. Although he regarded the method used by Sutton and Dimsdale as 'bogus' it is clear that those workers took great care to follow the effects of their inoculations, and they described in detail the normal course of events. For example, Dimsdale described painful axillae as a 'pleasing symptom' which 'foretells the near approach of the eruptive symptoms', which themselves were another sign of 'favourable progress'. The eruptive fever appeared by day eight – 'slight remitting pains in the head and back' (Dimsdale, 1769, pp. 31–2). It is also clear that there was a good local lesion. For example Baker described Sutton's method and remarked that there was 'constantly and invariably a large pustule' (Baker, 1766, p. 12). Sutton himself described the development of a clear vesicle, and regarded the failure of this to develop further as an 'unfavourable' sign, and stated that the febrile symptoms lasted from day nine to day eleven (Sutton, 1796, pp. 104–16). Chandler, in describing his use of the Suttonian system stated 'From the seventh day to the nineth or tenth day I expect my patients to begin to complain a little . . . in a day or two from their first beginning to complain the pustules seldom fail to appear' (Chandler, 1767, pp. 32–3). So it is clear that a favourable outcome (i.e., mild but effective) of the Suttonian inoculation was a well-developed vesicle accompanied by involvement of the axillary lymph-nodes and a mild but noticeable constitutional disturbance. We now know that immunity to diseases such as polio, diphtheria, and tetanus can be induced by the injection of killed virus or de-toxified toxins (toxoids) and we should have no hesitation in concluding that the methods popularized by Sutton and Dimsdale would have stimulated the immune system even in the absence of a generalized eruption.

In contrast the variolous test used by Jenner to test the immunity produced by previous exposure to cowpox had a much milder effect than that described by the variolators. Unfortunately Jenner gave very few details but the common result was usually described as inflammation or inflorescence which subsided by about the fifth day. One astute observation by Jenner, also noticed by some of the early variolators, was that the reaction following the challenge with smallpox often developed more quickly in those in which immunity had developed (Jenner, 1798, Case IV, p. 13). As noted above this feature had also been seen by Pearson. This accelerated anaphylactic reaction is now recognized as indicating previous exposure. The most significant and detailed account of the variolation of Pead and Barge by Henry Jenner had already been quoted (*see* pp. 63–4). These results demonstrated in a quite unequivocal manner that Pead and Barge were immune. The account showed at the same time the validity of the variolous test by the fact that 'regular' smallpox was produced in an unvaccinated control. Crookshank also regarded Jenner's use of the variolous test as unsatisfactory and this view was echoed in the Dissentient Appendix to the Royal Commission. All these critics believed that cowpox exerted at best only a temporary non-specific effect against smallpox and insisted that there was no practical basis for Jenner's belief. According to Creighton 'This disease [cowpox] was fancifully represented as an amulet or charm against smallpox, by the idle gossip of incredulous persons who listened only to the jingle of names' (Creighton, 1889, p. 33). Creighton also gave an account of how he believed that cowpox exerted its temporary effects. He suggested that cowpox:

caused a swelling and obstruction of the absorbent glands . . . and to that extent made them incapable . . . of taking up and passing into the lymphatic circulation another virus . . . Let us suppose that the glowing end of a cigar be firmly applied to an infant's arm; an eschar and an indurated sore will result which may be called cigar-pox. Let the variolous test be tried and there is every reason to expect . . . that the result will be the same as after cowpox . . . the cigar-pox is in its pathology just as relevant to the smallpox as the cowpox is (Creighton, 1889, pp. 149–50).

Variolation was illegal by the time Creighton was writing but had he tried the experiment it would have failed.

Quite apart from the interpretation of the variolous test these critics also thought that the bulk of the evidence presented by Jenner was insufficient to substantiate his main claim that cowpox protected against smallpox. However, I think that it is fair to conclude that the evidence in the *Inquiry*, though not extensive, was sound and probably sufficient to justify his main claim.

Jenner's briefly stated claim that the protection provided by cowpox was lifelong did not excite any immediate comment. It was not mentioned by Pearson or his correspondents. However, Haygarth's friend, Percival of Manchester, in a letter to Jenner wrote, 'But a larger induction is yet necessary to evince that the virus . . . renders the person who has been affected with it secure during the whole of life' (Baron, 1838, 1, p. 157). I suspect that here we have a glimpse of Jenner the dreamer. He knew that variolation did not always protect against smallpox, and that second attacks of smallpox sometimes occurred. So he ought to have been prepared for occasional cases of smallpox in people who had had cowpox or been vaccinated.

The claim that cowpox originated from horse grease received almost universal criticism. In 1805 Fraser revealed that Jenner had discussed this idea with Woodville before publishing the *Inquiry* and that Woodville had suggested that the idea should be dropped (Fraser, 1805). Pearson's comments on the theory perhaps summed up the most reasonable attitude:

> . . . this conclusion has no better support than the coincidence in some instances of the prevalence of the two diseases in the same farm, and in which the same servants are employed among the horses and cows. This assertion stands in need of support from other observations (Pearson, 1798, pp. 83–4).

Jenner's evidence was only circumstantial, and he was unable subsequently to produce any more certain evidence, and he gradually dropped this theory. However there was a germ of truth in the idea and vaccines were to be introduced from horsepox; these circumstances will be described in Chapter 12. Creighton, who was writing at the same time as Crookshank and did not know that the unpublished manuscript of 1796 had been discovered, assumed that the grease was not an important part of the original version, but in fact it was.

There was also considerable scepticism about Jenner's

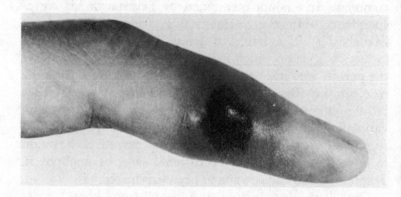

Figure 8 Accidental human cowpox, 1973. The patient had been successfully revaccinated only thirteen months previously (Author's Collection)

claim that people could have second and third attacks of cowpox. Pearson wrote of this 'I find that most part of professional men are extremely reluctant in yielding their assent to this fact. Some indeed, reject it in the most unqualified terms' (Pearson, 1798, p. 44). On this point, and Jenner's related claim that those who had previously been infected with smallpox were still susceptible to cowpox, Pearson wanted to know whether the second attacks were less severe than the first. Human cowpox is so rare that the chance of a person being exposed to it a second time must be extremely small. However, there is every reason to believe that second attacks would occur if the opportunity arose, for this is the basis of revaccination. The patient shown in Figure 8, a colleague of mine, became accidently infected with cowpox virus only thirteen months after being successfully revaccinated. The cowpox infection was much more severe than the revaccination. The appearance of the lesion is remarkably similar to one of the cases investigated by Crookshank and reproduced in Figure 9. Second attacks presumably occur because the virus is placed directly into the most favourable site for replication and it by-passes the hosts' defence mechanisms. Such a person might be expected to be resistant to natural smallpox because that virus would have to enter via the upper respiratory tract and would have

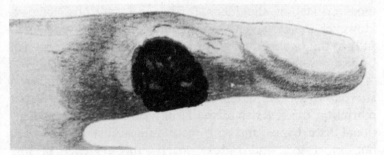

Figure 9 Accidental human cowpox, 1888. Figure 1 of Plate 2 from Crookshank's original account of the outbreak in Wiltshire. (Author's Collection, reproduced with the permission of the Editor of the *British Medical Journal*).

to run the gauntlet of the hosts' immunological and non-specific defence mechanisms before it could initiate infection. The problem of second attacks of cowpox, like the basic thesis that cowpox would protect against smallpox, was complicated by the concepts of 'true' and 'spurious' cowpox.

Jenner and his supporters found it most convenient to believe that spurious vaccine must have been used if the patient subsequently developed smallpox. Their reliance on this excuse probably inhibited a more rational study of such features as the effectiveness of, and duration of, the immunity following cowpox. However, despite this over-reliance on the concept Jenner was basically correct in his claims that cows were infected by types of 'cowpox' which did not protect against smallpox. Pearson obtained evidence of different bovine infections. His correspondents included a cowman who knew the cowpox 'which was described to be a very different disease from the common inflammations and eruptions which produced scabbed nipples' (Pearson, 1798, p. 29). Pearson accepted this and stressed that care should be taken to ensure that the correct type of cowpox was used (*ibid.*, p. 90). In a letter which Pearson published Jenner also explained his fears that people might inoculate 'putrid pus' instead of cowpox. These patients when variolated would then get smallpox, thus leading to 'injurious' conclusions (Pearson, 1798, p. 101). Creighton and Crookshank were most critical of the idea of true and spurious cowpox. However, Jenner's views on the subject were not presented fully in the *Inquiry*, and as the subject is a complex one it will be dealt with fully in Chapter 10.

The general acceptability of cowpox as a preferred alternative to variolation depended on such factors as the mortality, the severity of the local lesion and any constitutional disturbance, and on its communicability. Critics were not impressed, and rightly so, by the evidence of low mortality. The evidence on which this claim was made was based on very few cases and Pearson suggested that evidence from one or even two thousand cases should be sought before such a claim could be justified (Pearson, 1798, p. 66). However, his correspondents confirmed Jenner's claim that deaths had not occurred from natural cowpox, and Pearson suggested that the extra data would confirm Jenner's belief. Pearson also stressed the importance of determining what effect inoculated cowpox would have on those 'under the particular circumstances of Pregnancy; Age; Teething; Peculiar morbid states; Peculiar healthy states or Idiosyncrasies; and certain Seasons of epidemical States'.

In his *Inquiry* Jenner had said that John Baker (Case XVIII), who had been inoculated with material one remove from a horse, could not be variolated because he 'was rendered unfit for inoculation [variolation] from having felt the effects of a contagious fever in a work-house'. Later, in his next pamphlet he admitted in a footnote 'that the boy unfortunately died of a fever at a parish work-house' (Jenner, 1799, p. 23). Both Creighton and Crookshank criticized Jenner severely for withholding the truth. They pointed out that it was strange that Jenner, as an experienced practitioner, should refer to a contagious fever without making a diagnosis. They concluded that Baker had died from erysipelas as a direct result of the vaccination. It is possible that the vaccination led directly to Baker's death, but it is equally possible that he really was killed by a work-house fever. If Baker had been killed by erysipelas, this would have been caused by the contaminating bacteria rather than by the actual vaccine virus, and given the level of understanding at the time would have been unavoidable. However, this episode is a good example of how Jenner's tendency to provide insufficient information was used by critics who were ready to find fault at every opportunity.

There was much discussion about the appearance of the cowpox lesion and the constitutional disturbance it produced. To a certain extent the problem was caused by Jenner's ambiguity in this matter. He overstressed the similarity between the local lesion of cowpox and that of inoculated smallpox. The similarity between the general symptoms of cowpox and inoculated smallpox, namely the axillary involvement and general indisposition, was probably worth stressing. However, he demonstrably erred in stressing the similarity between the lesions of cowpox and inoculated smallpox because the similarity was in fact very slight. The pustule produced in natural smallpox is not a very alarming thing in itself; neither the size of the lesion nor the degree of inflammation would excite particular comment. However, there is a difference between the lesion produced by natural smallpox and the local lesion of inoculated smallpox. Jenner described and illustrated the lesions on the arm of Hannah Excell which 'so much resembled, on the 12th day, those appearing from the insertion of variolous matter, that an experienced Inoculator would scarcely have discovered a shade of difference'. However, this claim is not borne out by Jenner's engraving of Excell's arm which is reproduced in Figure 7 (p. 62). This showed three lesions very similar to those produced by blood-borne smallpox virus, i.e. those of natural smallpox or of the secondary lesions of inoculated smallpox. They are quite different from the local lesion of inoculated smallpox. This dissimilarity was soon to be noticed, first by Woodville, and used as a means of distinguishing between inoculated smallpox and vaccination. Briefly the differences were that the vaccination lesion had an even, almost circular, outline and it enlarged in a regular manner, whereas the local lesion of inoculated smallpox had a jagged irregular outline and tended to spread in an irregular manner with the development of small satellite pustules. Jenner's other two engravings of vaccination, one of which has been reproduced as Figure 6 (p. 61), and the engraving of accidental cowpox reproduced in Figure 4 (p. 59), all show lesions quite unlike those of inoculated smallpox. The direct comparison can be seen in Figure 10 which was used to illustrate the monograph by Paytherus (1801) and which is typical of other illustrations published by for example, Ballhorn and Stromeyer (1804), George Kirtland (1802), and George Pearson (1802).

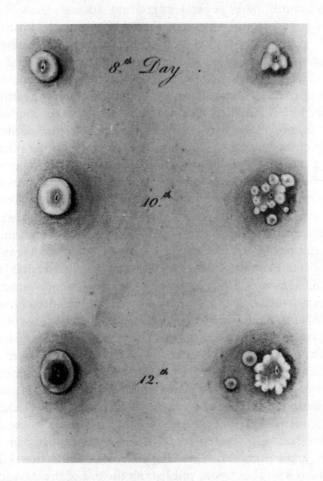

Figure 10 A comparison of the local lesions of vaccination (left) and variolation (right) at various times after inoculation, from Paytherus, (1801). (Liverpool University)

The degree of severity to be expected was apparent from the section of the *Inquiry* in which cowpox was described. Jenner mentioned that the lesions became ulcerated, and that they often healed slowly and frequently became phagedenic (Jenner, 1798, p. 5). When discussing individual cases the relative severity was also obvious. For example, William

Stinchcomb had 'several corroding ulcers', and Sarah Nelmes had a 'large pustulous sore'. Consequently those who were led to believe that the lesions of inoculated cowpox resembled those of inoculated smallpox were to find the actual lesions unexpectedly severe. On the other hand, those who appreciated that cowpox could produce a relatively severe lesion thought that this might reduce its acceptability.

It is not clear why Jenner overstressed the similarity between cowpox and inoculated smallpox. I suspect that it was part of the reasoning that led him to invent the term variolae vaccinae for cowpox, namely that cowpox and smallpox must be related and so there must be similarities. In any event it was the severity of the cowpox lesion which attracted attention. Sims, writing about a case which might well not have been true cowpox anyway, referred to it as the 'most loathsome of diseases' and commented that this 'circumstance entirely overlooked in Dr Jenner's account, appears to be itself a formidable objection to its introduction' (Sims, 1799). Lawrence, a veterinary surgeon, wrote of cowpox as 'filth and nastiness' (Lawrence, 1799), a phrase which was later to be echoed by Crookshank. After the publication of the *Inquiry* Jenner started another series of vaccinations which was curtailed because the lesions were troublesome. He had to treat them with caustic, and relayed this information to Pearson. Pearson of course knew that Jenner had also treated some of the cases reported in the *Inquiry*, and replied, 'On telling Dr Woodville that I had been anxious about your publishing the use of the caustic he replied "that would have damned the whole business". Be assured that if the practice cannot be introduced without the caustic . . . it will never succeed with the public' (Baron, 1838, I, p. 315).

Later Crookshank was to emphasize the loathsomeness of cowpox, and drew up a list of quotations from Jenner's and Pearson's descriptions of cowpox. In this list words and phrases such as 'sores', 'several corroding ulcers', 'large pustulous sores', 'painful sores as large as a sixpence' etc., were emphasized in bold type (Crookshank, 1889, 1, pp. 352–3).

From our present position there are two comments that can be made about these descriptions of early cowpox. The first is that it is not possible to determine whether any tendency of the vaccine to produce untoward effects was due to the inherent properties of the virus, or whether it was caused by the presence of contaminating bacteria. The second, and most important, point is that despite the comments made about the apparent severity of the lesions, they would not be regarded as being particularly severe by today's standards. I think that the relative severity of the lesion was over-emphasized by many of the early workers, perhaps because they were using an unknown virus from the 'brute' animal and were worried that the local lesion was more severe than that of human smallpox which they knew well. The opponents of vaccination would naturally tend to over-emphasize the severity. That Crookshank's reaction to the loathsomeness was in fact hypocritical will be shown in Chapter 10. I have been allowed to use in Figure 11 a photograph which has already been used in colour by a leading authority to show a typical primary vaccination. The caption stated 'the local lesion consists of a pearly pustule, mounted on a red indurated base. The pustule may be haemorrhagic . . . Constitutional disturbance may be considerable' (Emond, 1974). The similarity between the present-day vaccination and the engravings shown in Figures 4, 6, 7, and 10 is very obvious and will be discussed further in Chapter 13. For the present we can say that those who expected cowpox inoculation to look like inoculated smallpox would be surprised, but that the severity should not have surprised later workers who were familiar with the appearance of vaccination. However, as will be pointed out later both Creighton and Crookshank had particular reasons for emphasizing the severity.

Jenner's attempt to equate smallpox and cowpox was severely criticized at the end of the nineteenth century. To

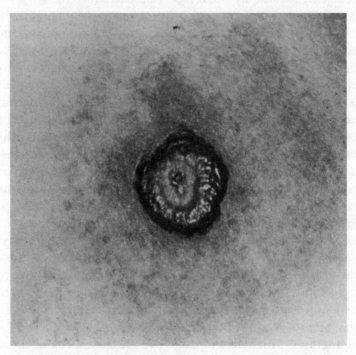

Figure 11 Typical primary vaccination, 1974. Reproduced from the colour transparency published by Dr R.T.D. Emond. Compare with Figures 6, 7, and 10. (Reproduced with the permission of Dr Emond and Wolfe Medical Publications).

some extent the problem was aggravated by the efforts of Jenner's biographer, Baron, to equate a generalized pustular disease of cows (cattle plague) with smallpox in man. Creighton was incensed by Jenner's use of the term *variolae vaccinae* – smallpox of the cow. He referred to this repeatedly throughout his *Jenner and Vaccination* as Jenner's 'master stroke', 'startling novelty', 'blushing invention', etc. He believed that Jenner's use of the term was the crucial factor in a deliberate attempt to mislead the medical profession. I think that there is a much more innocent explanation for Jenner's motive. He knew that his vaccine did not cause smallpox in humans. Therefore (despite his speculations on the topic), it couldn't really be smallpox. He had convinced himself that cowpox protected against smallpox. Therefore it must be related to smallpox. So what better name to use than smallpox of the cow, or, since it was to be used in a learned treatise, variolae vaccinae?

However, to Creighton, cowpox was not even related to smallpox. 'It was not a nice disease, and Jenner ought to have known why the dairy folk had instinctively called it a pox' (Creighton, 1889, p. 42). Creighton believed, as had Benjamin Moseley, one of Jenner's earliest critics, that cowpox was really modified syphilis, and had already devoted a whole book to the topic (Creighton, 1887). Crookshank also stressed the similarity between cowpox and syphilis (Crookshank, 1889, 1, pp. 461–7). With arm-to-arm vaccination there was a possibility that syphilis might occasionally be transmitted along with the vaccine. However, this possibility was over-emphasized by some critics, and of course there is no relationship between cowpox and syphilis.

So in summary Jenner's claim that cowpox protected against smallpox, although based on relatively slender evidence, was a reasonable claim to make. His suggestion that the immunity was life-long was unwise, and his claim that cowpox originated from a disease of horses was based on rather circumstantial evidence. The claim that vaccination was a safe alternative to variolation was also reasonable although he caused some confusion by making ambiguous references to the effects of vaccination. He was severely criticized for suggesting that second attacks of cowpox could occur, and in particular for suggesting that there was true and spurious cowpox, but in fact he showed an accuracy and insight that many of his later critics lacked. Although, as we will see, the first extensive trials of vaccination were still to be made, and the nature of the first widely-used vaccines is still in doubt, Jenner's *Inquiry* is a remarkable account of the introduction of vaccination.

I have repeatedly referred in this and other chapters to the criticisms of Jenner which were made by Crookshank and

Creighton. Jenner had many critics but these two have been singled out for two reasons. Firstly, they wrote at the end of the nineteenth century and so had the whole of that century's data to draw on. This they did very extensively even if they interpreted it in a rather subjective way. Secondly, they were the most learned and influential critics, and minor critics such as Tebb and Pickering drew both inspiration and information from them. Consequently it might not be out of place to say something about Crookshank and Creighton here.

Edgar M. Crookshank (1858–1928) was Professor of Comparative Pathology and Bacteriology at King's College, London. He was a dresser with Lister, and later studied with Pasteur and Koch. In 1886 he published his *Manual of Bacteriology* which was well-received and went through five editions. In 1887 he investigated an outbreak of cowpox in Wiltshire and published an account of it in July 1888. In this paper he quoted Jenner's work without criticism, and described cowpox without any indication that he regarded it as particularly severe. This outbreak prompted his historical investigations and led to the discovery of Jenner's un-published manuscript, and the publication of his *History and Pathology of Vaccination* in 1889. There is a certain inconsistency about the *History*. After claiming Jesty's priority for the first cowpox inoculation, and describing the development of apparently successful vaccines from cowpox and horsepox Crookshank finally concluded that neither of them 'exercise any specific protective power against human Small Pox'. The great value of the *History*, now itself a collector's item, is that it reproduces many of the early inaccessible pamphlets.

Unlike Crookshank, Charles Creighton (1847–1927) was most reluctant to accept the germ theory of disease. He was a graduate in both arts and medicine and spoke most European languages. According to Bulloch, himself a medical historian of note, he was 'the most learned medical scholar of the 19th Century' (Bulloch, 1927). He had a character defect which made him 'totally unfitted' for medical practice and instead he spent over thirty years studying medical history in the British Museum. There he wrote his *History of Epidemics in Britain*. This is still regarded as a classic work and a major source of reference and has been reprinted with added biographical information on Creighton (Creighton, 1965). 'The real tragedy of Creighton's life was connected with his views on cowpox and vaccination.' The tragedy to Bulloch was that it led to Creighton being ostracized by the conservative medical profession and becoming associated with the extreme elements of the antivaccination movement. The tragedy was also that Creighton missed the opportunity to prepare what could have been the most objective biographical and scientific analysis of vaccination that has ever been published.

After the publication of the *Inquiry* Jenner tried more vaccinations. Although he gave no details he said that he tried to inoculate cowpox without success. He had only limited success in November 1798. He inoculated two people with material obtained from a farm at Stonehouse in Gloucestershire. They both had relatively severe reactions but they both resisted variolation (Jenner, 1799, pp. 28–32). The virus was supplied to Mr Darke who vaccinated the Rev. Colborne's family, and two accounts of these vaccinations were published. One by Hughes, who had attended the children, gave detailed accounts of the results of the vaccinations which do not seem particularly severe. Of the five people vaccinated, three had lesions which cleared up in about nine days. Miss E. Colborne repeatedly rubbed off the scab which aggravated the lesion and delayed healing. However, 'although the arm undoubtedly teased her, [she] ate her food, and played with her sisters as usual the whole time'. The fifth patient had efflorescence surrounding the lesion which still had not disappeared by the eighteenth day and the scab did not separate until the twenty-ninth day. Again according to Hughes it 'was so little troublesome that he went on with the usual business'. When tested by variolation two of the patients had an accelerated local reaction and the other three had very mild smallpox (Hughes, 1799). They were variolated only seven days after vaccination, at which time specific immunity would only just have begun to develop.

The other account of the Colborne vaccinations by Thornton recounted hearsay evidence which he called 'authentic information'. According to this the children suffered severely from 'violent inflammation and alarming ulcerations in the arm' (Thornton, 1799).

So 1798 ended without any unequivocal confirmation of Jenner's main claim. The next significant events were to take place at the Smallpox and Inoculation Hospital in London. These events were to lead to the widespread use of vaccine and to a still unresolved controversy concerning the identity of the vaccine which was used.

7

The Jenner-Woodville Controversy

The London Smallpox and Inoculation Hospital was founded in 1746. As the name suggests it had a dual function, but it was not until about 1751 that regular variolation was practiced there. From 1752 to 1768 the number of patients variolated steadily increased from about 100 to over 1,000 per year. The location of the hospital was changed three times, both to provide increased accommodation and because of pressure from the local population which believed that it would be a source of infection. By 1750 the hospital had three houses, one for smallpox cases, one for the preparation of variolated patients, and one to which those variolated were transferred after inoculation. In 1752 the hospital was transferred to Cold Bath Fields, St Pancras, where it occupied a building with room for 130 beds and was set in its own extensive grounds. In 1798 the physician in charge was William Woodville, who had been appointed in 1791 (Figure 12). Woodville (1752–1805) obtained his MD degree in Edinburgh where he was a favourite pupil of William Cullen. He was in practice, first in Cumberland then in Denbigh, until coming to London in 1782 where he was appointed physician to the Middlesex Dispensary. He had a particular interest in medical botany which was then an important branch of medicine at a time when many medicines contained plant extracts. On his appointment to the Smallpox Hospital he laid out extensive gardens in the grounds in which plants of medicinal interest were grown. Woodville published his

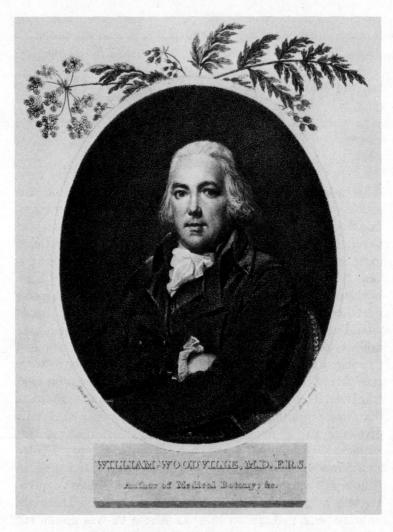

Figure 12 William Woodville, physician to the Smallpox and Inoculation Hospital in London. From an engraving by Bond. (Reproduced by Courtesy of the Wellcome Trustees).

Medical Botany in four volumes between 1790 and 1794. This great work, which described and beautifully illustrated the plants used to prepare medicines, was also published in two posthumous editions. Woodville's other great contribution to medical literature was his *History of the Inoculation of the Smallpox in Great Britain* to which reference has already been made. This was intended to be a two-volume work but only the first was published. This covered the subject up to 1768, and the second volume was abandoned at the proof stage when Woodville became involved in the vaccination controversy.

Obviously Woodville did not believe that his job required him to defend variolation against possibly better alternatives and he was very eager to investigate Jenner's claims. His first book on the subject '*Reports of a Series of Inoculations for the Variolae Vaccinae or Cowpox*' was published in May 1799. Although he did not believe that cowpox was derived from horse grease he thought that Jenner's 'other facts and observations concerning its effects upon mankind are not less valid and important' (Woodville, 1799, p. 9).

At the end of January 1799 Woodville heard of an outbreak of cowpox at a large dairy in Gray's Inn Lane, London, and went there with a friend of Jenner's, Thomas Tanner, a veterinary student, who confirmed the diagnosis. Woodville then invited a group including Sir Joseph Banks, George Pearson, and Robert Willan to see the animals and also a milkmaid who had been infected from them. The lesions were examined and compared with those in Jenner's *Inquiry* and, as Woodville wrote in his letter to Jenner, 'and upon comparing *your figure* with the disease, it was allowed by all to be a very faithful representation' (Baron, 1 pp. 307–8). Woodville started his series of vaccinations at the Smallpox Hospital on 21 January and wrote to tell Jenner of the circumstances on 25 January in the letter just mentioned. Between 21 January and 10 March he vaccinated 200 people and did another 400 or so between then and the publication of his *Reports* in May.

Woodville recorded his results in considerable detail. He gave an account of the vaccination of each of the first 200 patients which included the date on which they were vaccinated, named the donor, described the progress of the lesion and any constitutional disturbance, and noted the effect of variolation. Figure 13 reproduces Woodville's account of the vaccination of Ann Bumpus (Case 25), Woodville's most famous patient to whom greater attention will be paid in the next chapter. Woodville also summarized his results in a long table which showed the age of each vaccinee, the donor of the vaccine, the number of days of

---

TWENTY-FIFTH CASE.

Ann Bumpus, aged twenty years, was inoculated Feb. 6, with the matter of Cow-pox,
taken from the arm of Sarah Butcher. The
appearances of the inoculated part in this
girl's arm, correfponded in every refpect
with thofe ftated in Weft's cafe.   8th day.
                                        She

51

She complained of head-ach.   10th day.
Pain of the head and loins; fhiverings.
11th day. Two or three puftules appear
upon her face.   13th day. Pains continue;
more puftules appear.   15th day. No complaint: the puftules were counted and found
to be 310, refembling thofe of the Smallpox.   17th day. Complains of fore throat.
19th day. Puftules drying.   22d day. Inoculated with the matter of Small-pox, but no
inflammation was produced by it.

Figure 13 Woodville's account of the vaccination of Ann Bumpus, pp. 50–1 of Woodville's *Reports* (1799). (Liverpool Medical Institution).

illness and the number of pustules which developed. Part of this table showing the results of some of Woodville's first vaccinations is shown in Figure 14. Woodville had intended to publish an account of his first 200 patients earlier but was unable to do so. So he took the opportunity to list in the same tabular form the results obtained with another 310 patients although no details were given in the text. He also mentioned that he had vaccinated another 100 or so, but they were people who would not let their names be published, or whose

116

	Age Years.	Months	Days of Illnefs.	No. of Puftules.
From BUTCHER to				
Jewel	20	—	2	0
Bumpus	20	—	6	310
Weft	21	—	5	20
W. Hull	11	—	4	200
H. Hull	13	—	1	8
S. Hull	8	—	2	120
From JEWEL to				
Fifk	—	4	4	40
Reed	15	—	5	70
From S. PRICE to				
Pedder	—	11	5	40
Hoole	—	5	5	102
Hickland	—	6	3	300
Morton	—	9	7	200
From FISK to				
Davy	—	3	1	3
Murrell	—	7	4	20
From BUMPUS to				
Dixon	19	—	4	174
W. Walker	—	11	0	0
Cummins	—	3	0	0
Elliftone	—	3	2	0
Dunn	—	8	3	0

Figure 14 Part of the extensive Table in Woodville's *Reports*. This section shows the results obtained with the virus used to vaccinate Ann Bumpus. (Liverpool Medical Institution).

lesions were not sufficiently advanced for the results to be included.

One thing immediately apparent both to Woodville and to anyone reading his account was the fact that many of his patients developed generalized eruptions; in fact about 60 per cent did so. This came as a complete surprise to both Woodville and to Pearson who was helping him because Jenner's *Inquiry* had stressed that inoculation of cowpox did not cause eruptions. On 15 February Pearson wrote to Jenner, 'You will be astonished at our talking of eruptions, but it now appears in Dr Woodville's cases that as many have eruptions on the body as have them only on the inoculated parts' (Baron, I, pp. 313–14). Of the first seven patients inoculated from the cow on 21 January four had a generalized eruption, as did two of the five inoculated on 24 January from Sarah Rice the dairy maid. Because the eruptions occurred in the first patients inoculated directly from the cow Woodville believed that they were a natural consequence of inoculated cowpox. According to Pearson it was he who first suggested to Woodville that the eruptions might have been smallpox. Woodville did consider this possibility but discounted it on two grounds. Firstly, he had used newly-ground lancets and thought he could not have introduced smallpox that way. Secondly, though he had also variolated some of the vaccinees, he believed he had taken vaccine from them before the variolation had affected them (Woodville, 1799, pp. 137–9). These people had been variolated because at the start of the trials Woodville did not know whether the vaccinations would be successful. Because the patients were accommodated in the Smallpox Hospital and were 'constantly exposed to the infection of the Smallpox' he took the precaution of variolating them. However, in spite of appreciating the need to take these precautions, the possibility that any of his patients might have acquired natural smallpox did not occur to him at that time.

Woodville noted that when he used material from the secondary pustules as vaccine it had a greater tendency to produce pustules. Thus the general proportion of patients with pustules in his trials was about 60 per cent but out of 62 who were inoculated from secondary pustules 57 developed a generalized eruption (Woodville, 1799, p. 152). He noted that there was a lesser tendency to produce a generalized eruption if he took material from the local lesion and from people with only a local lesion. However, patients with generalized eruptions continued to occur sporadically throughout his trials. Although he did not think that the virus generated in the local lesions could produce natural infection in the same way that smallpox could, he did think that when cowpox produced a general eruption 'the exhalations they send forth are capable of infecting others in the same manner as the Small Pox' (Woodville, 1799, p. 154). Despite his belief that cowpox caused the eruptions he still concluded that it was a safe alternative to variolation but only if the virus was 'taken from those in whom the disease appeared in a very mild form'.

Despite the confusion over the production of generalized eruptions Woodville's *Reports* made two important points. Firstly, he was the first to publish an account which stressed the differences between the local lesions of cowpox and inoculated smallpox. As explained earlier Jenner had over-stressed the similarities. However, according to Woodville cowpox 'assumes a form completely circular, and it continues circumscribed, with its edges elevated and well defined . . . whereas that which is produced from variolous matter either preserves a pustular form or spreads along the skin and becomes angulated and irregular or disfigured by numerous vesiculae'. He also remarked on the different character of the cowpox scab which was harder and of a different colour (Woodville, 1799, pp. 146–7). These differences were soon to be confirmed by other investigators (*see,* for example, Figure 10) and can be made use of in attempts to identify the viruses used in some of the early vaccines.

The second point was that Woodville was the first to show that cowpox could be inoculated back into the cow after being taken from a human vaccinee. From Sarah Rice, the dairy maid infected naturally in the original outbreak, the virus was used to vaccinate Crouch (Woodville, 1799, Case 10, pp. 34–5). Virus from Crouch was used to infect a cow at the Veterinary College and virus from the cow was used to start a series of vaccinations beginning with Cases 40–42 (*ibid.*, pp. 62–4). It is interesting to note that Crouch did not have a generalized eruption, but that the three people inoculated from the cow had 300, 105, and 350 pustules.

The concern expressed by many at the severity of the lesions described by Jenner has been described in the previous chapter. However, the local lesions produced by Woodville's vaccines caused no alarm. According to Woodville 'the inoculated part has not ulcerated in any of the cases which have been under my care, nor have I observed inflammation to occasion any inconvenience, except in one instance' (Woodville, 1799, pp. 155–6). Jenner was puzzled by this tendency of the London virus to produce milder lesions and was to speculate that it might be due to differences between the London air and that in the country.

If taken at face value the results of Woodville's trials represent an extensive confirmation of Jenner's claims, and certainly the general acceptability of vaccination was founded on Woodville's experience and on the experience of those who received vaccine from him and Pearson. However, Woodville's results have not and cannot be taken at face value. The most controversial feature of Woodville's results was of course the development of generalized pustules in so many of his patients. In the short term this led to a disagreement with Jenner which was made public in an acrimonious exchange of pamphlets. In the long term it led to a debate concerning the identity of the vaccines which were developed at the Smallpox Hospital, which still continues.

It is clear that in the early months of 1799 there was an amiable exchange of information between Jenner in Gloucestershire and Woodville and Pearson in London, and in February Pearson sent some vaccine to Jenner from the arm of Ann Bumpus, one of Woodville's patients. Jenner sent his preliminary results with this vaccine to Woodville in time for them to be summarized briefly in Woodville's *Reports*. It had behaved exactly as the 'true uncontaminated cowpox'. The term 'uncontaminated' was to be at the heart of the disagreement.

Jenner published his second pamphlet *Further Observations on the Variolae Vaccinae* at about the same time that Woodville published his *Reports*. Jenner's main purpose in publishing the *Further Observations* was to deal in greater detail with the problems of true and spurious cowpox, and to print letters from some people who supported his general claims. However he also included an account of his use of the Bumpus vaccine on two children, one, a relative Stephen Jenner. Jenner was puzzled by the accounts of generalized eruptions in those vaccinated at the Smallpox Hospital. We can be sure he would be looking for pustules because the letter from Pearson which accompanied the vaccine was the one quoted above in which he told Jenner of the eruptions at the Smallpox Hospital. On the eighth day after Stephen Jenner was vaccinated 'a few spots now appear on each arm. . . . They are very small and of a vivid red colour.' By the tenth day the spots on the arm had disappeared, but three appeared on the face. Two of these had gone by the eleventh day and the other was barely perceptible. On the thirteenth day Jenner noted the similarity between the local lesion and that illustrated in his *Inquiry*. In the second patient, James Hill, the inflammatory area around the lesion was studded with minute vesicles and the local lesion healed slowly because the scab was accidentally knocked off. Virus from Hill was supplied to Henry Hicks who vaccinated eighteen people without any generalized eruption developing (Jenner, 1799, pp. 57–61).

From March 1799 onwards vaccines provided by Pearson from Woodville's stock were widely used and the results obtained will be discussed in Chapter 9. It was from this time that Jenner's disagreement with Pearson started, as with

Woodville, over the cause of the generalized eruptions.

In August 1799 Dr John Ring, the influential London physician, published a letter in the *Medical and Physical Journal* asking for clarification concerning reports that the vaccine inoculation caused generalized eruptions (Ring, 1799). Jenner replied to this personally in August saying 'from the time I first heard that pustules similar to the variolous had appeared among the patients inoculated there with the vaccine virus, I strongly suspected, from a coincidence of circumstances, that by some imperceptible avenue the variolous virus might have crept into the constitution at the same time'. This letter was not published until 1801 when Ring included it, along with the original letter, in his *Treatise on Cowpox* (Ring, 1801, pp. 71–9). The first indication the general public had that Jenner considered Woodville's patients to have smallpox came early in 1800. Pearson wrote a short note for the *Medical and Physical Journal* in which he discussed the tendency of cowpox to produce a generalized eruption which 'resembles very much if not exactly, some varieties of smallpox' (Pearson, 1800a). Jenner's reply was published in the same issue. He explained that he had very occasionally seen 'a few scattered pimples about the body' but stressed that they were quite unlike smallpox pustules. He concluded, 'I very much suspect, that where *variolous pustules* have appeared, *variolous matter* has occasioned them' (Jenner, 1800a). He returned to this theme in his third pamphlet *A Continuation of Facts and Observations relative to the Variolae Vaccinae or Cowpox* (Jenner, 1800b). He pointed out that the result of Woodville's trial 'differs essentially from mine in a point of much importance'. He went on to express his belief that the eruptions in Woodville's patients could not have been produced by '*pure uncontaminated Cow Pox virus*' and stated his opinion that the eruptions were caused by 'the action of the variolous matter which crept into the constitution with the vaccine' (Jenner, 1800b, pp. 7–8). He then described experiences with vaccines from London in a way which some think was a deliberate attempt to deceive.

Jenner received the Bumpus vaccine in February 1799, and obtained a different strain of cowpox from Kentish Town, London, in June 1799. He gave both strains to his friend and colleague Dr Joseph Marshall. Marshall reported his results with the Bumpus strain in a letter dated April 1799. Jenner, however, published the letter without a date in his *Continuation* and inferred that the results described the use of the Kentish Town strain (Jenner, 1800b, pp. 11–15). Marshall's letter of course was written before Jenner had received the Kentish Town strain and the results described in the letter referred to the Bumpus strain which Marshall had used on 107 patients. Two or three had erysipelatous lesions and 'in only one or two of the Cases have any other eruptions appeared than around the spot where the matter was inserted'. Jenner then printed a second letter from Marshall written in September 1799 by which time he had vaccinated 296 people with the Bumpus strain and 127 with the Kentish Town strain. Marshall was aware that Woodville's vaccines were producing eruptions in the Smallpox Hospital and was looking for them himself, but 'in all my Cases there never was but one pustule, which appeared on a patient's elbow on the inoculated arm, and maturated' (Jenner,, 1800b, pp. 17–18). Despite the confusion over Marshall's letters, the results were not affected because Marshall stressed the similarity of the results obtained with the two vaccines.

Woodville issued a reply in his *Observations on the Cowpox* which was published in July 1800. In his preface, a dedication to Jenner, he mentioned that in his attempts to refute Jenner's claim that the vaccines were contaminated with smallpox he was 'unable to avoid a certain degree of recrimination'. After dealing with Jenner's rather pompous claim to great experience he went on to discuss the Bumpus strain. He pointed out correctly that the vaccine had been taken from a patient who had 310 pustules, all of which suppurated, yet it did not produce pustules when used by

Jenner, Hicks, and Marshall. So, Woodville argued, it could not have been contaminated with smallpox virus (Woodville, 1800, pp. 7–11). In simple terms Woodville was probably correct, but the possibility that the Bumpus strain was contaminated and the extent to which it was typical of Woodville's strains will be discussed in the next two chapters. Woodville spotted Jenner's mistake over Marshall's letters and the Kentish Town lymph. He pointed out that Jenner was incorrect to suggest that Marshall's first 107 patients had been vaccinated with this strain. In a footnote he suggested that this 'very striking misrepresentation' must have been a mistake and not a deliberate attempt to mislead (Woodville, 1800, pp. 8–11). One ironic feature of this episode was that Woodville obtained a sample of the Kentish Town strain from Jenner and tested it on three patients at the Smallpox Hospital 'on one of whom about 100 variolous-like pustules were produced' (Woodville, 1800, pp. 19–20).

Woodville mentioned that although eruptions continued to occur sporadically in the Smallpox Hospital neither he nor unnamed colleagues (probably Pearson) had seen any tendency to produce eruptions in private practice. So although he still denied that his vaccines were contaminated he began to 'admit that they [the generalized eruptions] have been and still continue to be the effect of some adventitious cause, independent of the Cow-pox' and 'began to suspect that there existed some peculiar cause which rendered the patients under the vaccine inoculation in the Hospital more liable to pustules than others' (Woodville, 1800, pp. 18–19). Since the same vaccines and techniques were used in the Hospital and private practice he concluded that 'the only cause remaining to which the frequent occurrence of pustules . . . can be rationally referred, is the variolated atmosphere of the Hospital, which these patients were necessarily obliged to inspire during the progress of the Cow-pox infection' (ibid., pp. 20–1). One exception to the tendency not to produce eruptions outside the Smallpox Hospital was noted by

Woodville. More than 100 vaccinations were done in a village outside London during a smallpox epidemic, and one in five of those vaccinated had eruptions (*ibid.*, p. 22).

Once Woodville had realized that cowpox should produce only a local lesion and that the eruptions had been caused by smallpox the dispute between him and Jenner was a rather narrow one concerning the way in which the infection was acquired. The dispute was examined by Thomas Paytherus, a friend of Jenner's, who published a pamphlet in which statements from Jenner's and Woodville's publications were reprinted and commented upon. He neatly summed up the main point of the argument 'The contest therefore between Dr Jenner and Dr Woodville is reduced to this point: – Whether the *Small-pox by variolating* [i.e. contaminating] *the virus of Cow-pox, has crept into the system, and been the cause of the variolous-like pustules at the Hospital,* or whether, as Dr Woodville asserts, they have been occasioned by exposure to the *Variolated Atmosphere of the Hospital*?' (Paytherus, 1801, p. 23).

The way in which Woodville's patients became infected with smallpox is very difficult to determine even by close examination of his records. The nature of the viruses taken from an inoculation site would depend on whether the patient was inoculated with contaminated vaccine or whether the smallpox was acquired naturally, and would also depend on the timing of inoculation, natural infection, and sampling of the local lesion. In any event it was soon generally recognized that many of Woodville's patients did have smallpox and this view has never been seriously challenged. When Woodville appreciated this, together with the importance of taking material from those with a local lesion only, the proportion of his patients developing smallpox dropped to about ten per cent. However, the realization came after Woodville had completed the 510 vaccinations listed in the *Reports*. In fact the results obtained with the second 310 were worse than those in the first 200. For example in the first series 45 per cent had a local lesion only, 14 per cent had more than 100 lesions, and 1·5 per cent had more than 500 lesions. In the second series 39 per cent had a local lesion only, 21 per cent had more than 100 lesions, and 6 per cent had more than 500 lesions.

Woodville was correct to draw attention to Jenner's pompous claim to great experience in vaccinating. Jenner's actual practical experience of vaccination was very limited. Until he received the Bumpus strain in February 1799, it was limited to the few cases in the *Inquiry* and the rather unsatisfactory results with the Stonehouse strain. Consequently he was unable to supply vaccine to others until he himself had obtained virus from London. In contrast Woodville and Pearson distributed vaccines very widely. However, although Woodville's work set vaccination on a firm practical basis he inadvertently started a controversy which has not been resolved. When Ring in 1801 wrote that 'the Smallpox Hospital was the most unfit place in the Kingdom for the experiment' he thought he was commenting on the end of a controversy rather than the beginning. The problem concerns the nature of the vaccines which Woodville and Pearson distributed and was caused by the smallpox contamination. At the end of the nineteenth century, i.e. before it was realized that cowpox and vaccinia were not identical, there were three views on the identity of Woodville's vaccines.

1. One view was that cowpox had played no effective role in the development of either the immunity of Woodville's patients or of the vaccines which were distributed. It was believed that Woodville's original cowpox vaccines quickly became contaminated with smallpox virus, and that the immunity had been induced in effect by variolation. Consequently the vaccines which became so widely used on which the practical basis of vaccination was established were really attenuated strains of smallpox. Cowpox had nothing to do with it and consequently all Jenner's claims were void. The principal proponent of this view was

Crookshank who stated quite forcibly, '*I must repeat, the immunity was produced by SMALL-POX which was introduced into the constitution as a result of vaccinating in a variolous atmosphere or of employing contaminated lancets*' (Crookshank, 1889, I, p. 163). The two dissenting members of the Royal Commission, who were influenced by Crookshank also expressed the same view in their minority report (Royal Commission, 1898, pp. 365–8). They also stated that 'Woodville's lymph passed exclusively through those suffering from smallpox' (*ibid.,* p. 366). This is not so. Although he learned the danger of passing material from the secondary pustules, Woodville sometimes took virus from those with just a local lesion. For instance many of those vaccinated in the first series which was started from the cow on 21 January were given material which had gone through two successive patients both of whom had only a local lesion; these were Butcher (Case 17) and Jewel (Case 27) at the second and third remove from the cow (Figure 15, *see* p. 106). Later, at the seventh remove, vaccine lines passed through Pluckrose (Case 159) or J. Wall (Case 154) both of whom had only a local lesion. Similarly the vaccine started from Sarah Rice on 24 January went through some patients who had only a local lesion.

Crookshank and his supporters were correct in one important respect. Because of the presence of smallpox in so many of Woodville's patients, however they may have acquired it, his results could not be used to lend any weight to Jenner's claim that cowpox protected against smallpox. Consequently the strength of Jenner's claim still rested on his own early cases.

2. The second view was that of Creighton, who did not believe that smallpox played a significant role in Woodville's trials. He believed that Woodville had been lucky enough to select and propagate a mild strain of cowpox virus which produced less severe effects, but that basically its true relationship was to syphilis rather than

to smallpox (Creighton, 1889, pp. 106–19). The apparent protective effect of the cowpox used by Woodville was caused by a combination of the bogus variolous test, the concurrent naturally-acquired smallpox, and the 'cigar-pox' phenomenon discussed earlier.

3. The third view could be said to represent the pro-Jenner lobby. In their opinion Woodville succeeded in obtaining true cowpox from the infected animals. Although many of his patients became infected with smallpox the effective agent in the vaccines which emerged and which were so widely used was the original animal poxvirus which had outgrown the smallpox. This was the view expressed briefly by McVail (1896) and at some length by the Royal Commissioners (1898, pp. 315–33).

As explained in Chapter 1, present-day strains of cowpox virus can be differentiated from modern vaccine strains and modern analyses of the problem have to be made with this in mind. In 1965 Peter Razzell suggested that the vaccine which emerged from Woodville's trials was attenuated smallpox. This view has recently been presented again and in greater detail (Razzell, 1977a) but unfortunately Razzell did not take the opportunity to discuss alternative derivations which I believe would explain the facts equally well. Razzell's view is essentially a modern interpretation of Crookshank's view.

The only way information can be obtained on the possible identity of Woodville's vaccines is by analysing the detailed reports which were left, in the light of present-day know-ledge. The one episode on which attention has always been focused was the derivation and use of the Bumpus strain. This strain is particularly important because it forms a direct link between Woodville and Jenner. In addition some believed it to be representative of all Woodville's vaccines, and in particular believed that it formed the bulk of the vaccine used in the early years of the nineteenth century. Having outlined Woodville's experiences we can now examine the Bumpus strain in more detail.

8

Ann Bumpus

As I have briefly described in the previous chapter, Pearson sent a sample of Woodville's vaccine to Jenner on 15 February 1799. It was enclosed with the letter quoted earlier in which Pearson told Jenner of the eruptions in the vaccinees at the Smallpox Hospital. Pearson's letter gave no information about the source of this strain but Woodville later identified it precisely. 'The matter sent was taken from the arm of Ann Bumpus, who had three hundred and ten pustules all of which suppurated' (Woodville, 1799, p. 141). As we have seen Jenner, Hicks, and Marshall used the Bumpus strain on a total of 316 patients between mid-February and September without any smallpox pustules developing.

The pedigree of the vaccine from the cow to Bumpus can be traced with the aid of Figure 15. Virus from a cow was used to vaccinate Jane Collingridge (Case 6) and six other people, three of whom developed generalized eruptions. On the eighth day after her vaccination Collingridge's lesion was perfectly circular and had a 'lemon-coloured tint'. By the eleventh day the edge of the lesion 'was beset with minute confluent pustules' but by the thirteenth day it was 'subsiding and forming a scab'. Collingridge was variolated on the other arm five days after being vaccinated, and a generalized eruption started to appear on 3 February (i.e. thirteen days after vaccination and eight days after variolation). She developed 170 pustules 'in no respect differing from variolous pustules of the mild sort' (Woodville, 1799, pp. 27–8). Virus was taken from

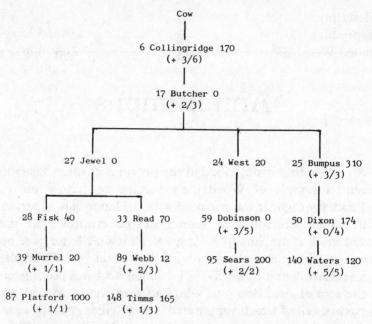

Figure 15 Chart showing part of the early pedigree of one of Woodville's main vaccines. The number preceding the name is Woodville's case number. The number following the name gives the number of pustules that patient had. The fraction under the name indicates the number of additional patients vaccinated with the same material (denominator) and the number of those who developed a generalized eruption (numerator).

Collingridge's local vaccination lesion on 30 January and used to vaccinate four others. So the virus was taken four days before the eruption started to appear. In many respects the circumstances in which Collingridge was vaccinated resembled those of Bumpus whose case is discussed in detail below. Virus from Collingridge was used to vaccinate Sarah Butcher. Butcher (Case 17) did not develop a generalized eruption but two of the other three did. Virus from Butcher was used to vaccinate a total of six people, namely Jewel on 5 February, Bumpus and West on 6 February, and three others on 8 February. Of these, all but Jewel developed a generalized eruption. Butcher was variolated, but only after the vaccine material had been taken from her. Woodville's description of the vaccination of Ann Bumpus (Case 25) is reproduced in Figure 13. By the time Bumpus was vaccinated Woodville was giving a relatively short description of events unless something unexpected happened. Bumpus developed a generalized eruption. The first two or three pustules appeared on day eleven (17 February) and by 21 February she had 310 pustules. Bumpus was not variolated until 28 February, long after the eruption started (Woodville, 1799, pp. 50–1).

It is generally assumed that Ann Bumpus developed small-pox. However, another, admittedly less likely, alternative is that she had generalized vaccinia. This is a complication of vaccination which is caused by the virus spreading from the local lesion through the blood to other parts of the body with the consequent production of a generalized eruption virtually indistinguishable from smallpox. It is now very rare and how much more common it was in the eighteenth century is impossible to determine. However, if Bumpus did have generalized vaccinia then smallpox played no part in the development of the vaccine sent to Jenner, and the views of Crookshank and Razzell would not be valid. The possibility that generalized vaccinia might have occurred should be considered whenever a patient developed a smallpox-like eruption in the week or so following vaccination.

If we assume that Bumpus had smallpox we then have to try to determine whether her vaccination lesion contained smallpox virus on the day the sample for Jenner was taken. Unfortunately it is not possible to determine with certainty whether she was infected by contaminated vaccine, or naturally by the upper respiratory tract from one of Woodville's patients. It should be remembered however that she was vaccinated with material from Butcher who did not have a generalized eruption and who presumably did not have smallpox. So if Bumpus's smallpox was acquired by inoculation, the smallpox virus would have already been contaminating Woodville's lancet. The eruption in inoculated smallpox developed from about the ninth day onward

(Figure 16), whereas Bumpus's eruption started from day eleven and on that day there were only two or three lesions. Consequently her eruption started a little late for it to be regarded as a typical case of inoculated smallpox, although given case-to-case variation it is possible that she was infected by inoculation. In naturally-acquired smallpox the eruption usually developed from days fourteen to fifteen onward. So if Bumpus had been infected in this manner the most likely time for her to have been infected was in the two or three days before she was vaccinated. Again there is case-to-case variation and it would have been possible for her to have become naturally infected at the time she was vaccinated or even a day or two after that. Nothing is known about the precise arrangement of the patients in the Smallpox Hospital. However the eruptions of some of Woodville's vaccinees started at about the time that Bumpus may have become infected, and may have been the source of infection. For example Buckland's eruption (Case 3) started on 1 February, Collingridge's (Case 6) on the 3rd Payne's (Case 4) and Bunker's (Case 9) on the 5th, Brown's (Case 14) on the 6th, Harris's (Case 8) on the 7th, and Talley's (Case 13) on 8 February. In addition to these we might also possibly consider infection from any of Woodville's smallpox patients.

Pearson's letter to Jenner was dated 15 February but it is not known whether the virus was taken from Bumpus on that day or earlier. However, the important point to note, as previously mentioned by McVail (1896) and the Royal Commissioners, is that Bumpus's eruption did not start until 17 February on which day she had only two or three pustules. Consequently if Bumpus's smallpox had been acquired naturally I think it is extremely unlikely that her vaccination lesion would have contained smallpox virus on or just before 15 February. Robert Willan, the great dermatologist, discussed this question with specific reference to Woodville's practice in his *On Vaccine Inoculation* (1806). His conclusion was 'that fluid taken from the vaccine vesicle on the arm of a person affected with the variolous fever and eruption, and inserted into the arm of another person by a clean lancet produced the vaccine disease alone. Numerous experiments assure me of the correctness of this observation' (Willan, 1806, pp. 6–7). Although I think that a failure to transmit smallpox might not always occur, particularly in the case of severe smallpox, I think it would apply in the case of Bumpus at the crucial time, because her smallpox eruption had not started.

If Bumpus had been inoculated with vaccine contaminated with smallpox on 6 February her local lesion need not necessarily have contained smallpox virus on 15 February. Whether it did would depend on the relative amounts of the two viruses which were inoculated and on how the two viruses would interact in the lesion. I believe that the most likely outcome is that the vaccine would outgrow any contaminating smallpox. Cowpox (and also vaccinia) develops more quickly than smallpox both in humans and in experimental systems. Figure 16, taken from a paper by Hime (1896), shows how inoculated smallpox develops more quickly than natural smallpox and how vaccination develops more quickly than either. Consequently the smallpox virus would have to develop in the face of the host defence mechanisms which would have already been stimulated by the other virus. These defences would include the development of specific immunity provided by antibody as well as non-specific resistance provided by the production of interferon. From Figure 16 (p. 110) it can be seen that Hime considered immunity to start at the end of the second week after vaccination. However, the methods then available for measuring immunity were very crude and now antibody production can be detected as early as the end of the first week after vaccination. The increased temperature in an inflamed lesion can also be regarded as a defence mechanism. It is significant in this respect that smallpox virus will not replicate above $38.5°C$ whereas cowpox replicates at $40°C$.

If the vaccination lesion had been very heavily contami-

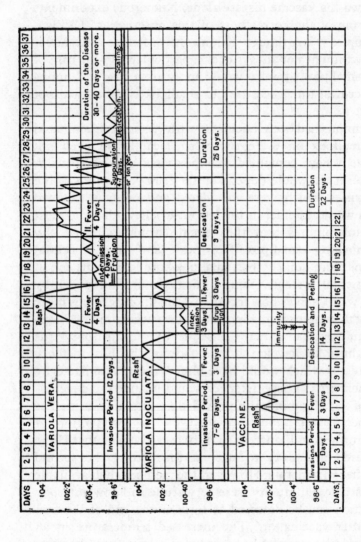

Figure 16 Chart showing the clinical course of natural smallpox (variola vera), variolation (variola inoculata) and vaccination. From Hime, (1896). (Author's Collection. Reproduced with the permission of the Editor of the *British Medical Journal*).

nated with smallpox virus, the vaccine would again have
outgrown the smallpox but might have taken longer to do so.
If this was the case we should have seen some evidence of this
in Bumpus and the people vaccinated from her. However,
there is no such evidence. As we have seen Woodville could
distinguish between the local lesions of vaccine and smallpox
but found nothing remarkable about Bumpus's lesion. In
addition the material used by Jenner, Hicks, and Marshall
did not produce smallpox. Consequently I think that it is
most unlikely that the vaccine taken from Bumpus and sent
to Jenner contained significant amounts of smallpox virus.

Could it have contained anything else other than the virus
Woodville originally obtained from the cow? There are two
other possibilities. Razzell believes that Woodville's vaccines
were developed by the attenuation of smallpox virus, and
cites the Bumpus strain as a particular example of this
(Razzell, 1977a, pp. 22–39). Consequently, in this view, the
material from Bumpus was either vaccinia or smallpox in the
process of becoming vaccinia. However, there is no evidence
from Woodville's descriptions of the local lesions in
Collingridge, Butcher (who had no generalized eruption) or
Bumpus that this vaccine ever was predominantly smallpox.
Failure of the Bumpus vaccine to produce generalized
eruptions when it was out of the Smallpox Hospital was both
rapid and dramatic, and Woodville noted similar results with
his other vaccines. As we have seen, no rapid change took
place in pre-Jennerian times.

It is most important to appreciate what is implied by the
suggestion that vaccinia is attenuated smallpox. It does not
mean that vaccinia virus is smallpox virus acting in an
attenuated way. Attenuated virus vaccines are now quite
common. The best known perhaps are those used to prevent
polio and measles, but others are available. In all these cases
the attenuated virus strains are clearly recognizable as minor
variants of the appropriate parent. On the other hand
although vaccinia and smallpox viruses are immunologically
related members of the genus *Orthopoxvirus*, they are

otherwise quite distinct. Whatever previous generations may
have thought, these two viruses are different in very many
respects. Their biological behaviour is different (Baxby,
1975), there are differences in their protein composition
(Harper *et al.*, 1979), and there are even minor antigenic
differences between them (Gispen & Brand-Saathof, 1974).
All these differences mean that their DNA should be
different and this has been confirmed by recent analyses
(Esposito *et al.*, 1978; Mackett & Archard, 1979). Consequently if vaccinia was derived from smallpox virus it would
require not just attenuation of the characteristics by which
the two viruses are superficially differentiated but the general
transformation of one virus into another.

Experimental work with smallpox in humans has of course
been out of the question. However, some attempts have been
made to change the characteristics of smallpox virus under
laboratory conditions, and these experiments have shown
just how genetically stable smallpox virus is. For example,
two characters which enable laboratory workers to
differentiate between smallpox and vaccinia viruses are the
inability of the former to grow in the rabbit skin or at
temperatures above 38·5°C. In 1966 Dumbell and Bedson
managed with great difficulty to adapt two strains of
smallpox virus to grow on the rabbit skin. They did this by
first carefully adapting the virus to growth in rabbit cell
cultures. The following year, along with M. Nizamuddin,
they reported successful attempts to adapt two strains of
smallpox virus to growth at 40°C. This again was achieved
only with difficulty by subculturing the virus 44 times as the
incubation temperature was gradually increased from 37°C.
In all other respects the smallpox virus remained smallpox
virus, i.e. these workers succeeded in producing rabbit-
adapted or thermo-efficient strains of smallpox virus rather
than bringing about any other tendency to transform. For
smallpox virus to have become transformed to vaccinia
during the development of the Bumpus strain would have
required so many interrelated mutations, leading to the

production of an entirely different virus, that I think that it is most unlikely to have happened. Later, deliberate, attempts to produce vaccinia from smallpox virus will be discussed in Chapter 11.

The final possible identity of the Bumpus vaccine is that it was a genetic hybrid of smallpox and cowpox viruses. This origin for vaccinia in general was suggested by Bedson and Dumbell in 1967. They argued that smallpox and cowpox viruses between them possess almost all the characteristics of vaccinia and were able to produce hybrids in the laboratory with ease. Although a hybrid with the precise properties of vaccinia has not been produced, only a small number of hybrids has been isolated (Bedson & Dumbell, 1964).

A genetic hybrid could have been produced only if Bumpus's lesion had contained large amounts of both parental viruses. It is an absolute requirement for hybridization that both parental viruses should replicate in the same cell in order for the genetic exchange to take place. Because the cell is large compared to the discrete inclusions in which virus replication takes place, infection by more than one of each type of virus would be required to ensure that the inclusions integrated sufficiently to allow hybridization to take place. If hybridization did take place any hybrid formed would have to compete successfully with its parents, otherwise cowpox would again have been selected out. However, vaccinia would have advantages because it grows more quickly and is less susceptible to elevated temperatures than both cowpox and smallpox viruses. Consequently a hybrid with the properties of vaccinia would outgrow its parents.

As discussed above, the probability is that if Bumpus's vaccination lesion was contaminated with smallpox (which is itself doubtful) then the contamination must have been slight. Consequently I do not think that suitable conditions for hybridization were set up. It is interesting to note that the idea of hybridization occurred to both Woodville (1799, p. 140) and Willan (1806, p. 7), who both discounted it. They were of course thinking of hybrid diseases and did not know that the diseases were caused by specific infectious agents which are themselves capable of genetic hybridization under suitable conditions.

Although the Bumpus strain was probably not a hybrid, some nineteenth-century vaccines may well have had such an origin. However, there are some objections to the idea that present-day vaccines may be hybrids and these will be discussed in Chapter 13.

In summary I would like to state my own opinions about the origins of the Bumpus vaccine. In its immediate effects, as described by Jenner, Hicks, and Marshall, it behaved in a way that came to be regarded as typical of vaccinia. If Ann Bumpus had generalized vaccinia, then smallpox would have played no part in the vaccine taken from her. If she had naturally-acquired smallpox it is most unlikely that her local lesion would have been contaminated at the time that the virus was taken from it. If it had been contaminated, then the degree of contamination was so low that hybrids would not have been produced, and the original virus would have outgrown the contaminating smallpox. Rapid attenuation of smallpox could not have occurred because the number of necessary interrelated mutations could not have occurred in the time available. Although it is theoretically possible for the Bumpus strain to have been derived by any one of the methods just discussed, I believe that the vaccine obtained from Bumpus was essentially the same that had been taken from the cow. Whether this was what we would now recognize as cowpox virus is more difficult to determine and will be discussed again in Chapter 13.

Apart from providing material for Jenner, Woodville made only limited use of the virus from Bumpus. It was used on 18 February to vaccinate two people, neither of whom had eruptions, and again on 24 February to vaccinate three more, one of whom had 174 pustules (Woodville, 1799, pp. 68–70). It is not possible to determine whether these five patients had been inoculated with a sample of the material which had been sent to Jenner, or whether fresh material had been taken on each occasion.

The Bumpus strain can be placed into the perspective of Woodville's trials by reference to Figure 15 (p. 106). As well as showing the pedigree of the Bumpus strain, the cases have been selected to demonstrate three particular features:

1. Some cases of what are presumed to be smallpox occurred sporadically throughout the series, with no attenuation occurring with respect to the number of pustules. For example Bumpus at third remove had 310 pustules, Sears at fifth remove had 200, Platford at sixth had 1,000, and (not shown) Hales and W. Goddenn had 500 and 650 pustules at the seventh remove.

2. Material from eruptive cases sometimes gave rise to non-eruptive cases, for example Collingridge to Butcher. The possible explanations of this are the same as those discussed above where virus taken from Bumpus, who had a generalized eruption, did not produce eruptions in those vaccinated by Jenner and Marshall.

3. Patients receiving vaccine from non-eruptive cases sometimes developed eruptions, for example Jewel to Fisk and Read, and Dobinson to Sears. The possible explanations of this are the same as discussed above where Bumpus developed an eruption after being inoculated with virus from Butcher who had no eruption.

It is difficult to estimate what effect the immunity induced by the vaccine had on the concurrent smallpox in Woodville's patients. Only one of Woodville's patients died. This was a baby with 80–100 pustules who had 'fits of the spasmodic kind' (Woodville, 1799, pp. 149–50), and it is not certain that smallpox was the cause of death. In all, 90 of Woodville's first 510 patients had over 100 pustules, 40 had over 300, and 21 had over 500 pustules. According to Dixon, deaths from smallpox can be expected to occur in those with 'discrete' smallpox, i.e. with 100 pustules but no confluent areas. In such cases the mortality is about two per cent. As the number of pustules increase and they become confluent on the face and/or arms the mortality reaches ten to twenty per cent (Dixon, pp. 6–7). Consequently the one death in Woodville's cases is considerably less than might have been expected, and it is probable that this reduction in mortality was caused by vaccination. Because vaccination progresses more quickly than natural smallpox the immunity which develops in response to the vaccine will have some effect on smallpox even if the vaccine is given in the early stages of the smallpox incubation period. Hopefully this vaccination will prevent the smallpox developing at all, and this may account for those of Woodville's patients who did not get eruptions. However, if vaccination in the incubation period fails to prevent smallpox in some patients it is generally recognized that it will reduce the severity of the illness, the number of pustules, and the overall mortality. Some of Woodville's patients had very few pustules. Of the first 510 patients, 90 had less than 10 and of these, 19 patients had only one or two pustules. Confirmed cases of smallpox with so few pustules have been recorded, and have caused fatal epidemics (Christie, 1969, p. 207). So these patients of Woodville's who had generalized eruptions can be thought of as cases of smallpox the severity of which had been reduced by the concurrent vaccination. Although this is the most likely explanation for the majority of patients, other explanations are possible and might well have applied to some patients. Some of the mild cases might have been second attacks of smallpox where the first attack had been incorrectly diagnosed as chickenpox. Some patients might have had generalized vaccinia. Some of the patients with very few pustules might have transferred the vaccine to other parts of the body by scratching; this is still common in human cowpox and would be more common in vaccinated people if they were not warned to avoid it. Some of the eruptions, whether extensive or not, might have had nothing to do with either vaccination or smallpox; they might have had concurrent skin complaints of any one of a number of types.

My overall impression of Woodville's practice is that of a series of vaccinations with a basically non-eruptive vaccine, which may have occasionally been contaminated with smallpox virus, and which was used in a contaminated atmosphere. In the important case of Ann Bumpus I think smallpox played little or no part. The behaviour of the other vaccines which originated from the Smallpox Hospital is best assessed by considering how they were used by their recipients both at home and abroad, and this will be the subject of the next chapter.

9

Other Early Vaccines

On 12 March 1799 George Pearson sent threads impregnated with vaccine to over 200 people, and this is an appropriate moment to have a brief look at the man who distributed them. George Pearson (1751–1828), like Woodville, studied medicine at Edinburgh and obtained his MD in 1773. After a short period in London and two years in Europe he returned to his native Yorkshire where he practiced for ten years. He became physician to St George's Hospital, London in 1787 where he taught chemistry as well as medicine. Whilst in Yorkshire he published a two-volume account of the springs in Buxton, Derbyshire, and was later to do research on carbonic acid, the discovery of calcium phosphide, and the chemistry of urine. He introduced the term 'nitrogen' into the English language.

His analysis of Jenner's *Inquiry* has been discussed earlier. The speed with which he assembled and published this analysis probably gives us some idea of his methods of working. In March 1799 he distributed vaccine widely and this and the publicity connected with it started the rift with Jenner. Jenner's nephew warned him that Pearson was about to undertake widespread distribution of vaccine 'by which means *he* will be the chief person known in the Business'. Jenner then suggested to his friend Gardner that 'some neatly drawn paragraphs [should] appear from time-to-time in the public prints . . . to keep the idea publicly alive that P. was not the author of the discovery' (Baron, 1838, 1, p. 320). In December 1799 the rift was wider. Pearson was instrumental in organizing the 'Institution for the Inoculation of the

Vaccine-Pock' the inaugural meeting of which took place on 2 December. The Duke of York was to be Patron and Pearson was to be the physician; there was no mention of Jenner. On 10 December Pearson wrote to Jenner to tell him of the project and offered him the post of 'extra corresponding physician'. Jenner expressed surprise that such a venture should have been initiated without his knowledge and concluded 'I must beg leave to decline the *honour* intended me' (Baron, 1838, I, pp. 360–2). When Jenner presented his petition to Parliament, Pearson gave evidence against Jenner and published his own critical account of the affair (Pearson, 1802). Jenner's unreasonable attitude has been emphasized even by such objective observers as Dixon, who suggested that Jenner was an impossible man to work with (Dixon, 1962, p. 267). This might have been the case but it is clear from just the bare facts of Pearson's actions that Jenner's patience must have been sorely tried.

It is interesting to note that although Woodville and Pearson co-operated in the Smallpox Hospital, Woodville gave no support to Pearson in his attack on Jenner's petition. Pearson lived until 1828 but little is heard of his interests in vaccination after about 1803. It is significant that Pearson made no substantial original contribution to vaccination. His published work on the subject, valuable though it is, consisted of analyses of the results of others and brief general defences of his views. I think that Pearson can reasonably be labelled as an opportunist who intended to enhance his reputation at both Jenner's and Woodville's expense.

Unfortunately it is not possible to identify the material distributed by Pearson. One of the basic principles of modern vaccine production is the conservation of the basic 'seed lot'. This is carefully selected and should receive only limited subculture. Batches of vaccine are produced from the seed lot after only a limited number of subcultures. This practice is aided by the fact that many large batches of seed lot material can be prepared and then preserved for long periods at low temperature. These methods, which restrict the number of subcultures which the vaccine goes through, ensure that no untoward changes occur.

In contrast the material distributed by Pearson should probably best be considered as a collection of closely related vaccines. Pearson had obtained his own strain of cowpox from Paddington in London early in 1799 and used this, as well as virus provided by Woodville, in his own practice. However, there is no record of the extent to which he used his own strain. Ring said that the vaccine he had obtained from Pearson was Woodville's because Pearson could not meet the demands from his own supply (Ring, 1801, p. 302). In addition to the vaccines described in his *Reports*, Woodville also mentioned that he obtained vaccine virus at various times from different cows and used it in the Smallpox Hospital (Woodville, 1800, p. 19).

Pearson's circular letter was dated 12 March 1799 and the threads would have been prepared in the week or so preceding that date. Examination of Woodville's *Reports* indicates that about 76 people were vaccinated between 25 February and 6 March, and material from them could reasonably be expected to be used. At this time Woodville was vaccinating an average of eight people with the virus from one donor. Consequently to load 200 threads he would have to obtain virus from perhaps 25 donors. Although it was known that vaccine could be preserved on thread it is possible that the threads were overloaded in an attempt to ensure that some virus would survive. So it is reasonable to regard 25 donors as the minimum number used. It is not known whether any virus was used which had been passed through Ann Bumpus. Virus from her arm was used to vaccinate two people on 18 February and five people on 24 February. From one of these latter cases virus was used to vaccinate six people on 3 March. The lesions of those inoculated directly from Bumpus would have started to heal by the time the threads were prepared but those on the arms of the people vaccinated on 3 March would have been suitable. At this early stage in the trials Woodville and Pearson believed that general eruptions were a natural consequence of cowpox so they would probably have taken virus from those with generalized eruptions as well as local lesions. However, following the practice of good variolators they would probably have avoided taking material from secondary pustules. Given the state of Woodville's practice at the time it was probable that some threads contained vaccine contaminated with smallpox virus.

We know very little of the men who received the threads. What is certain is that not all were medical men; some were clergymen. There were still political battles in the eighteenth and nineteenth centuries between physicians, surgeons, and apothecaries, and organized medical care for the needy was primitive. In these circumstances clergymen often helped and it was quite common for them to preach in favour of variolation in the pulpits and practice it in their parishes. So it was natural for some of them to be asked to try the new 'vaccine inoculation'. As we have seen Pearson had established a country-wide correspondence when he originally investigated Jenner's claims, so it is reasonable to assume that he would send threads to people who he believed to be experienced variolators but sympathetic to the new technique. In his circular letter Pearson asked them to report their results to him, which some did; others published their experiences in the *Medical and Physical Journal*.

The results obtained are not easy to interpret but in general can be placed into three categories:

1. Those in which smallpox appeared initially but which gave a characteristic vaccine appearance within very few passages.
2. Those in which a local lesion only was produced or which produced a very occasional case of smallpox.
3. Those in which the local lesion was accompanied by spots, pimples, rashes or single pustules.

Some recipients of Pearson's threads reported that it produced eruptions. Dr Redfearn, of Lynn in Norfolk, received his thread on 19 March and inoculated two people the following day. The first patient had 40 pustules which started to develop after eleven days. The eruption in the second patient also started on the eleventh day and was 'as copious as in the uninoculated smallpox'. The third patient was inoculated with virus taken from the local lesion of the first. This patient developed five or six spots on the face and hands. They 'made little progress in size and died away in the course of a few days' (Redfearn, 1799). Redfearn apparently abandoned his trial at this stage, which is unfortunate because it would have been interesting to see what happened during further transfers. One whose results were similar to those of Redfearn but who did carry out more vaccinations was T. M. Kelson, of Sevenoaks in Kent. He inoculated 'several' people with virus from one of Pearson's threads, but in only two did the virus take. One of these had a generalized eruption 'exactly like smallpox of the distinct kind'. People vaccinated from this patient had no generalized eruptions but all three vaccinated from one of these developed pustules. Use of this material at the fourth remove produced generalized eruptions in some of its recipients but thereafter no generalized eruptions were seen. The second of the two patients inoculated from the original thread had the infection 'in the mildest possible form'. This presumably means that there was a local lesion only, although this is not stated. A second series of vaccinations was started from this patient and none of the 100 or so vaccinees had a generalized eruption (Kelson, 1800).

The first vaccinations in Manchester were done in April 1799. Although the source of the vaccine was not stated it is probable that it came from Pearson. Nine people were vaccinated initially. The first became seriously ill and developed 1,600 to 1,800 pustules. The second had a typical vaccination response which healed by the eleventh day, but about 50 pustules appeared 32 days after vaccination; far too late for the vaccine to have been their cause. The vaccine failed to take in the third to sixth patients. Only a local lesion developed in the seventh and eighth patients both of whom resisted subsequent variolation. The ninth patient developed a few pustules around the local lesion. Five more patients were vaccinated with virus taken from the first patient. Two of these had generalized eruptions and the others either had no take or did not return for examination (Ward, 1799).

The difficulties experienced in assessing the results obtained by these early workers is perhaps exemplified by the results reported by Evans, of Ketley in Shropshire. He obtained virus in May 1799 from Addington who had one of Pearson's threads. He later obtained vaccine from Jenner but its precise identity is unknown; as it was obtained in June it would probably have been the Bumpus strain. In all Evans vaccinated 68 people, 39 of whom had eruptions; similar results were obtained with each vaccine. Interpretation of the results is difficult because according to Evans:

> At the same time I inoculated fifty patients with variolous matter . . . and whenever I had it in my power I inoculated one part of a family with vaccine and the other part with variolous virus (Evans, 1799).

A commendable but misguided attempt to conduct a controlled clinical trial.

In many respects the experiences of the above vaccinators are very similar to those of Woodville at the Smallpox Hospital. The possible identities of the vaccines which emerged from these trials are those discussed above in detail for the Bumpus strain. However, it is in instances such as those discussed above, where contamination with smallpox virus seems certain, that a hybrid origin was a real possibility.

Some correspondents reported that the vaccine produced a local lesion only, with perhaps an occasional case of smallpox. In October 1799 Pearson published a summary of the results obtained by himself and some of his correspondents. It was probably written in July or August and mentioned that 'In my private practice not a single case with eruptions resembling the smallpox has occurred in the last four months'. He also mentioned that the areola surrounding the local lesion was more marked than in variolation. However, he did not think the inflammation was serious and suggested that it could be referred to as erythema rather than erysipelas. As well as his own results he mentioned those of some of his correspondents who did not publish separate accounts, such as Mitchell of Chatham with no eruptions in 50 patients, and Harrison of Horncastle with none in about 100 (Pearson. 1799b). The Rev. Robert Holt, rector of Finmere in Oxfordshire, did publish his own account. His first patient had no pustules and according to Holt the 'appearance and progress were exactly similar to the description and beautiful plate given by Dr Jenner'. Holt vaccinated about 300 and mentioned three specific cases. One had a single pustule near the site of inoculation and the other two had eruptions resembling mild smallpox with about 100 pustules (Holt, 1799). Perhaps the simplest and most likely explanation of such results is that such practitioners were lucky enough to get a thread which was not contaminated with smallpox virus, and that the occasional case with eruptions was naturally acquired. Again however, any of the alternatives discussed above for Bumpus will apply here.

Most difficult to interpret are those cases in which the patient had spots, pimples, rashes, or single pustules, in addition to the local lesion. The difficulty arises because there is no certainty that these various effects had a single cause or that they were necessarily connected with the vaccination. The early vaccinators were usually very careful to distinguish between spots and pimples, which appeared early and regressed quickly, and a mature smallpox pustule. Similarly they distinguished between nondescript rashes and the generalized eruption of smallpox. It is possible that some of those who reported that the vaccine produced no generalized eruption might have missed or omitted to mention the production of spots or other rashes. Jenner's own observations have been dealt with above (p. 98). Pearson in 1800 summarized his own view. He estimated that spots, either singly or up to a dozen, occurred in about one case out of twenty or thirty. He described them as 'large, red, hard pimples' and they were of such a short duration and so unlike smallpox pustules that he did not class them as a smallpox eruption. He also mentioned occasionally seeing a rash similar to urticaria which appeared on about the fourteenth day (Pearson, 1800a).

One careful observer was the Rev. W. Finch, of St Helens in Lancashire. In November 1799 he obtained vaccine from Holt, whose results have already been described. Finch reported that he had vaccinated 714 patients. The first one had 'a small red spot under the left thigh. It produced no pustule'. One of the six children vaccinated from this first case had one pustule on the neck. Two boys inoculated at the third remove had local lesions only but at the next level one patient had two red spots which disappeared the following day without suppurating (Finch, 1800).

A most interesting comparison was made by Christian Stromeyer, the Court-Surgeon of Hanover. He had obtained one of Pearson's threads and also some vaccine from Jenner and compared their effects. 'This year we have inoculated 40 persons, as well with the vaccine matter received from Dr Pearson as that of Dr Jenner, all of which went properly through the disease.' The London vaccine produced 'pimples which disappeared in a day or two, but never that sort of eruption, repeatedly noticed in London, which so much resembles the smallpox'. He described the pimples as being similar to 'nettle fever'. Jenner's vaccine produced no eruption of any sort but did cause 'tedious' ulcers which took a long time to heal (Stromeyer, 1800). This is the clearest evidence, based on direct comparison, that different vaccines gave different results and it is extremely unfortunate that we don't know which of Jenner's strains was used. If it was the Bumpus strain it would provide strong circumstantial evidence that the Woodville/Pearson material should not be regarded as a homogeneous vaccine. John Ring also briefly discussed the rash which sometimes followed vaccination and thought it similar to a teething-rash (Ring, 1800).

These spots and rashes could have had many different causes. They could have been non-specific responses to the vaccine, the occasional infection caused by bacterial contamination or they could have been entirely unconnected with the vaccine. The occasional mature pustule such as that on the neck of Finch's patient could have been a secondary vaccine lesion transferred by scratching.

When attempting to assess the incidence and significance of spots and rashes we should also consider the distribution of spots, pimples and other skin eruptions in the unvaccinated in that relatively unclean age. The general level of health, hygiene, and nutrition was lower then and it is probable that a significant proportion of the population would have skin complaints of one sort or another. These first vaccinations were done in the very early days of modern systematic dermatology. One of the first rational attempts to classify skin disorders was made by Robert Willan in his *On Cutaneous Diseases*, published in parts between 1796 and 1808. He was awarded the Fothergillian medal of the Royal Society of Medicine for this work, and is often referred to as the Father of Dermatology. In this classic work and in his *On Vaccine Inoculation* (1806) Willan discussed the skin disorders which sometimes accompanied smallpox, variolation, and vaccination. He described a rash, *Roseola variolosa*, which sometimes accompanied smallpox, and which occurred during the eruptive fever. It occurred on the arms, breast, face, trunk, and extremities, and he estimated that it occurred in one in fifteen patients, particularly in those with delicate stomachs or skins (Willan, 1808, pp. 442–9). Such a rash with about the same incidence is described by modern smallpox authorities (Dixon, 1962, pp. 42–3; Christie, 1969, pp. 198–9). Willan also described the vaccinial equivalent, *Roseola vaccina*. This again occurred especially in those with delicate skins and was first seen about nine or ten days after vaccination and lasted no more than 48 hours (Willan, 1808, p. 450). In *On Vaccine Inoculation* (Willan, 1806, p. 10) he described an eruption which was found on the back and arms after vaccination.

Again there are modern equivalents. According to Christie a variety of rashes, both local and generalized, may occur after vaccination. 'As a rule they are macular, urticarial or non-descript in type' (Christie, 1969, pp. 224–5).

As well as considering such non-specific rashes caused by the vaccine, Willan also discussed other specific cutaneous diseases which might have been precipitated by vaccination. Although he did not consider that the incidence of such diseases was higher in the vaccinated than in the unvaccinated he listed those cutaneous diseases which had been diagnosed in vaccinated patients:

> The Lepra, the dry and the humid Tetter, the Prurigo, the chronic Nettle-Rash, and the Strophulus candidus, but more especially the Dandrift, the Favus, the crusta lactea, the scald-head, and the Ring-Worm (Willan, 1806, p. 82).

Razzell attached great significance to these various spots and rashes. If they occurred soon after a vaccine had left the Smallpox Hospital then they were an indication of smallpox becoming attenuated; if they occurred later, with an otherwise innocuous vaccine, they heralded the reversal of attenuation (Razzell, 1977a, pp. 48–54). However, the results are far too complex to be interpreted in this unambiguous way. Such an interpretation makes two big assumptions neither of which is necessarily justified. One is that the spots, etc. were a direct result of the vaccination. The other is that their appearance was unusually significant. I do not think that any great significance should be attached to such disorders. Their diverse nature was recognized at the time and their modern equivalents are well known. It is extremely doubtful whether their nature and incidence has any real bearing on the origin of the vaccines being used, except to introduce a source of confusion.

In some instances the early vaccines were implicated in smallpox epidemics. The two incidents usually quoted are a small epidemic in Petworth, Sussex, in October–November 1799 and a large epidemic at Marblehead near Boston, Mass.

in October–November 1800, in which 68 people died. Razzell attempted to trace a continuous line of vaccine from the Smallpox Hospital through Bumpus to Jenner and on to America, and from Pearson to Petworth. In this he assumed that the vaccines were identical, and most important he discounted the possibility that the smallpox could have been caused by anything other than the vaccine which had reverted to fully virulent smallpox (Razzell, 1977a, pp. 65–79). The Petworth epidemic was an embarrassment to both Pearson, who supplied the vaccine, and Jenner.

Pearson briefly sketched out the pedigree of the vaccine used at Petworth. It originated from virus taken from a cow in March 1799. This was after Woodville's series had been fully established and the source might well have been Pearson's own stock from the Paddington cow. Consequently its identity to Woodville's strains must be doubted. When first used it produced a few pimples 'not at all like the smallpox'. Virus from the first vaccinees was taken to Brighthelmstone (Brighton) by a Mr Keate who passed it on to Mr Barrett who vaccinated two children. From these other children were vaccinated. They all had eruptions and the local lesion had a ragged edge 'most resembling the variolous pustule'. Virus from these cases was sent to Petworth where it was used to vaccinate fourteen children (Pearson, 1800a). According to Dr Andre the vaccine 'produced a disease in every shape resembling the smallpox; the time of sickening, the symptoms, the eruptions and their maturation were the same' (Pearson, 1800b); at this time Pearson had been persuaded that cowpox could produce generalized eruptions and it was this incident which led Jenner to publish his view that 'where *variolous pustules* have appeared *variolous matter* has occasioned them' (Jenner, 1800a). It is not possible to determine with any certainty whether the vaccine used had contained some smallpox all the time, become contaminated after leaving Pearson, was an unstable hybrid or had reverted to smallpox.

The circumstances surrounding the epidemic at Marblehead are even more confusing and the link with Jenner and the Smallpox Hospital even more tenuous. Some of the vaccine used at Marblehead was provided by Benjamin Waterhouse. He had obtained it in June 1800 from John Haygarth who obtained it from Thomas Creaser who in turn had received it from Jenner. This was over a year after Jenner started using the Bumpus and Kentish Town strains, and it is impossible to determine with certainty the pedigree of the vaccine sent to Waterhouse. Waterhouse was the first person in America to try vaccination and he attempted to gain financially by establishing a monopoly. In an attempt to break this monopoly other vaccines were imported and by the autumn of 1800 there was a traffic in cowpox vaccine 'by non-professional persons' (Underwood, 1949). One such vaccine of unknown pedigree was imported into Boston by Dr Story just before the Marblehead epidemic started; an extract from Story's unpublished letter describing this was published by Razzell (1977a, p. 74). This vaccine was probably contaminated with smallpox and may well have caused some of the Marblehead cases (Baron, 1838, I, p. 388). If in addition the vaccine supplied by Waterhouse was responsible for some cases the possible sources of the small-pox were again the same as those discussed above. However, there is no certain evidence linking Marblehead in October 1800 with the Bumpus strain sent by Pearson to Jenner in February 1799.

The vaccines which became established from Pearson's threads would have the same potential origins as the Bumpus vaccine but need not necessarily have been identical to it. Many of Pearson's threads gave a local lesion only or occasional spots or rashes. These most likely contained the particular strain of cowpox with which they were loaded. The occasional single case of smallpox or smallpox epidemics, sometimes occurring many months after the vaccine had been originally distributed, were most probably caused by contamination with smallpox virus during later use. Some of Pearson's threads were contaminated with smallpox and

Kelson, Evans, and Redfearn probably used them. There is a real possibility here of a hybrid origin but as with the Bumpus strain the outgrowth of the original vaccine was the most likely result.

Throughout these analyses runs the possibility of contamination with smallpox. Some of the vaccines were contaminated initially, and some of those which weren't may easily have become contaminated at a later stage. Smallpox was endemic or locally epidemic in many areas and because vaccination was an experimental technique vaccination and variolation were often done at the same time. The description left by Evans and discussed above is the clearest evidence of the confusion this could cause. In addition Pearson when he sent out his threads urged that proof of the vaccines' efficacy should be obtained by variolating the vaccinees at a later date. Jenner was particularly concerned that contamination with smallpox would bring vaccination and himself into disrepute. The vaccinations at Petworth had been sponsored by Lord Egremont, and in a letter to him Jenner gave an example of how contamination could occur.

> Lancets are often carried in the pocket of a surgeon with smallpox dried upon them, for the purpose of inoculation. A gentleman some time ago sent a lancet here to have it charged, as it is called, with cow-pox matter: perceiving it stained at the point with some dried fluid it was sent back; when he immediately recollected that his lancet was prepared with the matter of the smallpox. What confusion might have happened from this; and how narrowly we escaped it! (Baron, 1838, I, p. 343).

The chances of contamination with smallpox in those early months must have been considerable. The further the separation from the time the vaccine was first established, in time space and number of users, the greater was the chance of contamination happening.

The vaccines originating from the Smallpox Hospital in February and March 1799, whatever their origin and whether homogeneous or not, were distributed very widely both in Britain and abroad. However, it is incorrect to assume as some have done that they were the only vaccines which were widely used at the time. The Kentish Town strain which Jenner passed on to Marshall has been mentioned previously. Jenner subsequently obtained this strain back from Marshall and vaccinated 'a considerable number with it'. He also mentions that he had 'dispersed it among others' but unfortunately gave no details (Jenner, 1800b, p. 22). However, we do know that it was sent to and used by Woodville (1800, pp. 19–20). Although this was after Pearson's threads were prepared, it is possible that the Kentish Town strain was distributed later.

Although it was customary to supply vaccine on threads to practitioners at a distance it was also customary for local practitioners to obtain virus directly from recently vaccinated individuals. In this way there would be a gradual diffusion of vaccines throughout the countryside. Although Jenner, his friends, and the Reports of the National Vaccine Establishment tended to refer to vaccines as coming from Jenner's original stock, this was probably a strategem intended to enhance confidence rather than an accurate statement. Certainly Jenner's original strains of 1796 and 1798 were soon lost so that the first strains he could have distributed were the Bumpus and Kentish Town strains. In 1800 he was using vaccine sent by Tanner, and in 1801 he was sent a vaccine from Italy by Sacco (*see* below). Although Jenner's actual practice was small and would probably not allow him to maintain more than one strain, he could have reintroduced other strains as he did the Kentish Town one by obtaining them from colleagues with more extensive practices. These would then have been passed on as 'Jenner's lymph'. The Royal Commissioners interpreted 'Jenner's lymph' to mean simply vaccine obtained from Jenner and this is a realistic assessment. They also commented 'We are not justified in assuming that an account of every new source of lymph was published, and there may have been others, it is impossible to say how many' (Royal Commission, 1898, p. 10).

Despite the understandable desire to use 'Jenner's lymph' or at least English lymph, attempts were made to find sources of vaccine abroad. Some claims, such as that by the Spanish expedition to South and Central America in 1803, should be viewed with caution (Baron, 1838, II, p. 80; Smith, 1974). Similarly the effectiveness of 'goat-pock' from Spain was not confirmed (Dunning, 1803). Waterhouse wrote to Jenner in May 1801 that he had apparently found 'kine-pox' in America, but three months later had to admit that he had been hoaxed by medical students who had inoculated the cows with vaccine (Waterhouse, 1801). However, there were authentic vaccines established on the Continent by Lafont in Salonica and in particular by Luigi Sacco in Lombardy. Sacco, 'the Jenner of Italy' was to become a target for Creighton, presumably because he rose from obscure beginnings to become one of the foremost vaccinators on the Continent. He found indigenous cowpox in Lombardy in 1801 and by October had written to tell Jenner that he had already vaccinated 8,000 patients 'several hundreds of these have since been subjected to the variolous inoculation and have resisted it' (Baron, 1838, I, 452–4). He described his early experiences in his *Osservazioni pratiche sull' uso de vajuolo vaccino* (1801), extracts of which were published in the *Medical and Physical Journal* (Sacco, 1802). He found that his vaccine did not cause eruptions and produced a less severe local lesion than the English strains. According to Creighton, 'He had not found them [phagedenic ulcerations] because he had not looked for them' (Creighton, 1889, p. 270). This strain was used very widely in Italy; by 1803 it was estimated that 90,000 vaccinations had been done with it (Noehden, 1803). Even more important is the fact that this vaccine was used very extensively outside Italy. In particular Sacco sent samples to Woodville and Jenner. Jenner, perhaps characteristically, passed it on to John Ring who wrote that 'it excited the genuine pustule, and, in my own practice, and in that of others is now spreading the vaccine preventive in every direction' (Ring, 1802). So we can certainly add Sacco's strain to those circulating in England in 1801. Sacco also sent a sample to Jean de Carro, an Edinburgh graduate originally from Geneva who had a large practice in Vienna. De Carro was certainly responsible for distributing Sacco's vaccine to the East. In a letter to Jenner he mentioned that 'the vaccine matter I originally sent to Bagdad, and which has propagated itself so widely was the product of the first experiment I made with the Cisalpine matter of Dr Sacco' (de Carro, 1803). There was also independent evidence of the widespread use of this vaccine. Whyte published a brief note on the introduction of this strain into Constantinople (Whyte, 1801), and Dr Christie from Ceylon wrote to tell de Carro that he had used vaccine 'from your Cisalpine stock which had reached us the preceding year by Bagdad Bassora and Bombay' (Christie, 1805). At about the same time that he was supplying vaccine to Constantinople, de Carro also supplied samples to Poland and Russia (Baron, 1838, 1, pp. 458–60), and although the strain is not identified it is possible that it was the same one.

So it can be seen that vaccines other than the Woodville/ Pearson strains were widely used. This fact has two important consequences. Firstly because it has never been suggested that they were ever contaminated with smallpox they provide independent and extensive confirmation of Jenner's claim that cowpox would protect against smallpox. This invalidates the criticisms of Crookshank, Creighton, and the Dissentient Royal Commissioners. Secondly the fact that they were so widely used tends to weaken the views of those such as Razzell who believe that virtually all of the early vaccine was supplied from the Smallpox Hospital and was attenuated smallpox.

Other vaccines were also introduced in the early years. These were established from infected horses and since they have a bearing on Jenner's 'grease' theory they will be discussed in Chapter 12. In the meantime we can turn our attention to another problem – that of 'true' and 'spurious' cowpox.

10

True and Spurious Cowpox

I have described in previous chapters how Jenner's concept of true and spurious cowpox was to cause a considerable amount of disagreement. Apart from its practical importance this subject is of interest because it shows us Jenner both at his most brilliant and at his most evasive. According to Creighton 'The cry of "spurious lymph" was the great excuse for the failure of cowpox to protect against smallpox, as well as for the ulcerous and bad effects of that infection itself.' To a great extent this is true. However, Creighton continued, 'It is unnecessary to show that the plea of "spuriousness" was a transparent piece of sophistry' (Creighton, 1889, p. 168). In fact Jenner's grasp of possible causes of spurious cowpox was, to use Dixon's words, 'quite masterly'. However, Jenner changed his ideas on the nature of spurious cowpox and this, together with the over-reliance on the excuse, was attacked with some justification by his critics.

Jenner's views on true and spurious cowpox were evidently not completely formulated at the time he wrote his *Inquiry*, and the brief mention in a footnote that care should be taken to select virus from true cowpox rather than from other bovine infections did not have the desired effect. I have described in Chapter 6 how Ingenhousz and others reported that smallpox had occurred in people who had previously been infected with what was thought to be cowpox. Because of this Jenner saw the importance of defining more clearly what he meant by true and spurious cowpox. This he did in his second pamphlet in a way which won him Dixon's praise.

However, before discussing this in detail it might be beneficial to outline what Jenner meant in general by the terms true and spurious cowpox. Creighton, Crookshank, and Pearson in his later critical period were to object to the use of these terms. To them cowpox was cowpox and the idea of true or false did not arise. The problem was caused by Jenner's use of the terms as a kind of shorthand for what he really meant. In other words true cowpox was that which was the *true* preventive against smallpox, whereas the spurious type was that which gave a *spurious* sense of security. The interpretation of his critics that what Jenner was describing was in any way true or spurious with respect to the cow was rather narrow.

In his *Further Observations* Jenner defined four sources of spurious cowpox (Jenner, 1799, pp. 4–5).

1st. That arising from pustules on the nipple or udder of the cow; which pustules contain no specific virus.

This was Jenner's recognition that there were bovine infections which when transmitted to man did not confer protection against smallpox. These various infections were gradually recognized by many during the nineteenth century. Discussion of these gives me an opportunity to describe briefly Crookshank's change of attitude over vaccination in general and Jenner in particular. Crookshank published his account of an outbreak of cowpox in 1888. It must have been what Jenner would have regarded as true, although Crookshank did not use the term, because subsequent attempts to vaccinate the infected farmworkers failed. Perhaps the most illuminating sentences in Crookshank's account were 'It must not be supposed that any sores or eruptions on the teats of a cow necessarily indicate cow-pox. It is necessary to bear in mind the existence of the following diseases of the teats of cows.' He then gave a brief account of diseases which Jenner would have regarded as spurious, although again the term was not used. These were chapped teats, blister-pock, aphtha epizootica, yellow-pock, bluish-pock, and warts (Crookshank,

1888, pp. 67–8). In his *History*, written after he had discovered what he believed to be the truth about Jenner, Crookshank wrote, 'Jenner was alone responsible for assuming the existence of two kinds of Cow Pox, a true and a spurious. And this assumption was extended in *Further Observations* to include not *one* but several kinds of so-called Cow Pox' (Crookshank, 1889, I, p. 278). Crookshank was also to change his mind in another respect as we will see later.

In his fourth pamphlet *The Origin of the Vaccine Inoculation* (1801) Jenner explained, perhaps with a little hindsight, how the discovery of spurious cowpox had been made. He was puzzled by the fact that smallpox occasionally occurred in those who were thought to have previously had cowpox. 'This for a while damped, but did not extinguish, my ardour; for as I proceeded, I had the satisfaction to learn that the cow was subject to some varieties of spontaneous eruptions upon the teats; that they were all capable of communicating sores to the hands of the milkers, and that whatever sore was derived from the animal, was called in the dairy the Cow Pox' (Jenner, 1801, p. 3). This same tendency to refer to a disease by a term which combines the name of the infected animal with the crude clinical description is still common and still causes confusion. However, in Creighton's opinion, 'Of all the many sly and impudent tales that Jenner told to the medical profession and to the public, the short sentence just quoted is the most sly and the most impudent' (Creighton, 1889, p. 163). However, Jenner was quite correct. The natural history of virus infections of the bovine teat is quite complex and has been investigated in detail by veterinary virologists from Bristol University (Gibbs *et al.*, 1970). They recognized five quite distinct viruses which produced localized teat infections, four of which occur naturally in Britain.

1. *Cowpox*. This of course is immunologically related to smallpox and so would not be placed in Jenner's first category of spurious. Circumstances in which it could act in a spurious way will be considered below when Jenner's

second and third categories are discussed. Bovine cowpox is now rare and its natural history, which is still not completely understood, will be considered in Chapter 12.

2. *Bovine Herpes Mammillitis.* This infection is much more common than cowpox but the causative agent, a herpes virus, was first characterized as recently as 1966 (Martin *et al.*, 1966). It does not infect man and so any lesions in people handling animals infected with this virus would be caused by contaminating bacteria and would fall into Jenner's second or third categories of spurious cowpox.

3. *Pseudocowpox* (Figure 17, p. 139). This infection is also called paravaccinia and both names suggest a relationship to vaccinia and cowpox. The infection is caused by a poxvirus, but one which belongs to a genus *(Parapoxvirus)* which is immunologically quite distinct from the genus *(Orthopoxvirus)* which contains smallpox, cowpox, and vaccinia. Pseudocowpox is extremely common in cattle and is easily transmitted to man where it produces a lesion not too dissimilar from cowpox. It is the prime candidate for Jenner's first category of spurious cowpox.

4. *Warts.* These are caused by papilloma viruses and the Bristol workers recognized two varieties, 'papilliform' warts and 'white nodule warts' (Figure 17). These are not transmissible to man so their possible involvement in spurious reactions would be the same as with bovine herpes mammillitis.

The Bristol workers also considered teat infections caused by vaccinia virus. This does not occur naturally but cases have been reported, particularly in Holland. The infection is transmitted accidentally to the cows from recently vaccinated people. The possibility that what we would now recognize as vaccinia could have existed naturally in Jenner's time will be discussed in Chapter 13.

Some of the above bovine infections are difficult to differentiate clinically. The confidence to make authoritative differential clinical diagnosis can only come from experience and from co-operation with a virus laboratory which can isolate the causative agent and so confirm or refute the clinical diagnosis. Jenner of course was working before such help was available, and if he made occasional mistakes this does not detract from the basic soundness of his idea.

Figure 17, supplied by Dr Paul Gibbs, is a remarkable photograph which shows a cow's teat which was naturally infected with 'true' cowpox and also two different kinds of 'spurious' cowpox. It is easy to imagine that someone could take material from the cowpox lesion and start a successful line of vaccine, and that someone else might take material from the pseudocowpox lesion and so fail to confirm the hypothesis.

In 1840 Robert Ceely, surgeon to the Buckinghamshire Infirmary, published a long paper on the natural history of cowpox in the Vale of Aylesbury. He accepted Jenner's concept of true and spurious cowpox and gave a brief description of different types of bovine infections which he regarded as spurious (Ceely, 1840, pp. 296–7). These included '*the Yellow Pock*', a pustular eruption on the teats and udders; '*the Bluish or Black Pock* [which produced] bluish, or black, or livid vesications on the teats and udders', and the '*White Pock*'. Of these three only white pock was said to infect humans, 'quickly causing vesications and deep ulcerations', and was frequently mistaken for true cowpox. According to Ceely it 'was often or almost always confounded by them [the milkers] with the true vaccine, and certainly not readily distinguishable in all its stages by better informed persons than milkers'. In addition to these infections to which Ceely gave specific names he also listed other bovine infections, one of which occasionally affected milkers.

We can now consider Jenner's second category of spurious cowpox.

2ndly. From matter (although originally possessing the specific virus) which had suffered a decomposition, either from putrefaction or from any other cause less obvious to the senses.

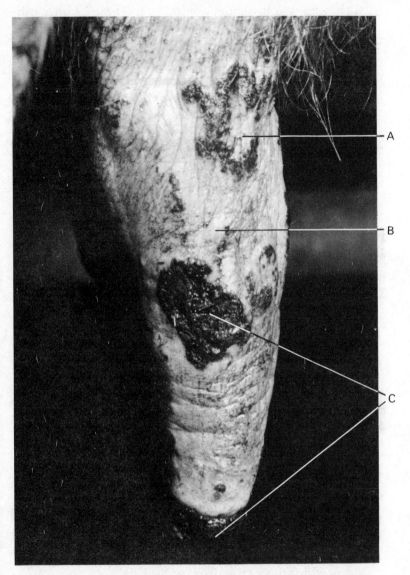

Figure 17 True and spurious cowpox on the same cow's teat. A = circinate lesion produced by pseudocowpox (i.e. spurious), B = white nodule variant of warts (spurious), C = scabbed lesions of true cowpox. From Gibbs *et al.*, (1970, 1973). (Reproduced with the permission of Dr Gibbs and the Editor of the *Veterinary Record*.)

This idea was in Jenner's mind at the time he wrote the *Inquiry* although it was not stated there in relation to cowpox. He discussed it in relation to ways in which errors could result from faulty storage of the smallpox virus which was to be used for variolation. It was this which Ingenhousz had criticized, and I can do no better than to quote Jenner's own words.

A Medical Gentleman . . . frequently preserved the variolous matter . . . on a piece of lint or cotton, which in its fluid state was put into a vial, corked and conveyed into a warm pocket; a situation certainly favourable for speedily producing putrefaction in it. In this state (not unfrequently after it had been taken several days from the pustules) it was inserted into the arms of his patients, and brought on inflammation of the incised parts, swellings of the axillary glands, fever, and sometimes eruptions. But what is this disease? Certainly not the Small-pox; for the matter having from putrefaction lost or suffered a derangement in its specific properties, was no longer capable of producing that malady . . . and many, unfortunately, fell victims to it [smallpox, when later exposed to the disease] who thought themselves in perfect security. (Jenner, 1798, pp. 56–8).

Soon afterwards, in a letter to Pearson, Jenner expressed his fears that the same thing might bring discredit down on vaccination. Nowadays great care is taken to prevent or reduce bacterial contamination both during the production and storage of vaccines. There is a strong possibility that the untoward effects of some of the early vaccines may have been caused by bacterial contamination. Jenner's third type of spurious cowpox was a variant of the second.

3rdly. From matter taken from an ulcer in an advanced stage, which ulcer arose from a true Cow Pock.

Here in modern terms we have a situation where bacterial contamination of the cowpox lesion has occurred. This, added to the effects of the host defence mechanisms, would reduce the virus content of the lesion. Consequently anyone inoculated with material from the lesion would be given either a mixture of virus and bacteria or perhaps just the contaminating bacteria alone. Although bacterial contamination of diagnostic specimens can now be controlled with antibiotics, failure to isolate virus from old lesions is not uncommon in virus diagnostic laboratories. Although bovine cowpox is relatively uncommon, I have been able to investigate an outbreak in collaboration with colleagues from Bristol. The outbreak first came to our attention when a farm worker became infected and cowpox virus was isolated from his lesion. However, by that time the lesions on the cows contained no virus. That their infection really was cowpox was confirmed by the results of serological studies on serum samples taken from the cows (Baxby & Osborne, 1979).

In the same paragraph in which he described Jenner's concept of spurious cowpox as 'quite masterly', Dixon wrote 'His [Jenner's] capacity to visualize the properties of a specific infective element distinguished from that producing the ordinary septic lesions and capable of loss through defective storage or not being present in a lesion too advanced, is quite remarkable' (Dixon, 1962, p. 284).

Jenner's fourth source of spurious cowpox shows him in a much less favourable light.

4thly. From matter produced on the human skin from contact with some peculiar morbid matter generated by a horse.

This is a reference to his grease theory. As explained in Chapter 5, Jenner believed that the source of his vaccine was an equine infection, but thought that it was only fully effective after it had been passed through the cow. He argued that direct inoculation of humans with equine material did not give satisfactory protection, i.e. it was spurious. This fourth category of spurious cowpox was solely and specifically concerned with equine virus. Yet within a few years vaccines were to be introduced directly from horses and were accepted and used by Jenner without him formally renouncing this fourth category. The subject of equine viruses is an important one and will be dealt with fully in Chapter 12.

There was another respect in which Jenner's views on spurious cowpox were inconsistent. Although he originally believed that the vaccine virus originated in horses, he did not say specifically whether it need have come from horses recently. In his *Inquiry* he gave accounts of some cases where he thought that the transfer from horse to cow had been recent. However, the majority of his cases of natural human cowpox were contracted from cows. No information was given about how or when the cows became infected from horses, which they must have been if his theory was correct.

This ambivalence is even more obvious when we consider such important vaccines as the Woodville/Pearson, Kentish Town, and Sacco strains. These strains were established from infected cows and there was never any suggestion that horses were involved in any way. Jenner, far from questioning the usefulness of these strains, accepted, used, and distributed them enthusiastically. One of two conclusions is possible. One is that, as his critics maintained, he conveniently dropped the idea that all spontaneous bovine infections were spurious. The other is that his original concept, although not clearly stated, envisaged that virus could be transferred from horse to cow at some remote time and that the virus could then be maintained in cows.

However, these were relatively minor problems compared to the extent to which the cry of spurious cowpox was used to excuse unwanted results. The exasperated Creighton posed himself a conundrum. 'When is the cowpox not the cowpox? Answer: (1) When it fails to protect from smallpox; (2) when it produces "morbid ulceration"' (Creighton, 1889, pp. 179–80).

There is not enough space to deal here with all the problems caused by cases of smallpox in people who had been vaccinated. Undoubtedly some cases were in people who had been given spurious cowpox. Willan analysed the problem and made two very sensible suggestions. Firstly he argued that failures of vaccination were only to be expected, particularly in view of the fact that in many cases it was being performed by untrained people. He pointed out that this should not be regarded as an argument against vaccination, and suggested that it should only be performed by competent practitioners. Secondly, in view of the fact that there might be uncertainty about the susceptibility to smallpox of those vaccinated in the crucial early years, he suggested that those who had been vaccinated before 1 January 1802 should be examined and revaccinated if necessary (Willan, 1806, pp. 46–9).

In fact two excuses were used for the failure of vaccination. If the fact that the patient had smallpox could not be denied, then it was argued that the vaccine must have been spurious. If the vaccine had been true, then the patient could not have smallpox but only something which might resemble it. In most cases where the vaccine was presumably true, any cases of smallpox which occurred on later exposure tended to be milder than they might have been expected to be, and in such cases a diagnosis of chickenpox was often made. In some cases reported to the *Medical and Physical Journal*, Bradley, the editor, offered his own judgement. For example Bevan reported an instance where a mother with smallpox had infected her two children, both of whom developed a mild eruptive disease which was diagnosed as smallpox. The children had been vaccinated and Bevan quite reasonably suggested that the vaccination had changed the system but not so completely as to prevent smallpox. To this letter Bradley added a footnote, 'We think that this eruption was not variolous' (Bevan, 1801). On another occasion Bradley published a letter from Stevenson on smallpox after vaccination under the running title 'Spurious Cowpox' (Stevenson, 1801). Stevenson objected to this and asked why Bradley had assumed that the vaccine had been spurious. Bradley published this second letter together with an explanation in which he admitted that he had sometimes used the term in too general and therefore incorrect a manner (Stevenson, 1802).

Some cases became *causes célèbres* because the patients were well known and in some instances had been vaccinated by Jenner himself. In such cases where Jenner was the vaccinator it could not be suggested that the vaccine was spurious, except of course by opponents of vaccination. One such instance was the case of the Hon. Robert Grosvenor, son of the Earl of Grosvenor. He had been vaccinated by Jenner in 1801 and had a perfect vaccination scar. In 1811 he had a very severe attack of smallpox and was attended by Sir Henry Halford and Sir William Farquhar. Although the attack had been very severe, they believed that the patient's recovery could have been due to the vaccination done in infancy and that Grosvenor would probably have died without it. A similar case was that of the son of Sir Henry Martin who was attended by William Heberden. The infection was perhaps not quite as severe as that of Grosvenor and Martin's life was never in danger. He had 'about one hundred pustules on the face and perhaps twice as many on the limbs, but the trunk was almost free', a perfect description of the distribution of the smallpox eruption. The boy recovered quickly and by the eighth day of the eruption the scabs were beginning to separate. The Board of the National Vaccine Establishment, which had its origins in the Royal Jennerian Institute, examined these cases and issued a pamphlet describing their findings. They concluded that Grosvenor had confluent smallpox and that Martin had a mild form of the 'distinct Small Pox'. They pointed out the usually fatal outcome of confluent smallpox and stressed that in these two cases the outcome had been modified by the earlier vaccination. They also described for comparison some examples of patients who had smallpox even though they had been variolated in the past (National Vaccine Establishment, 1811).

In the second decade of the nineteenth century, cases of smallpox in patients who had been vaccinated increased. Some of these were reviewed by Alexander Monro who also gave detailed accounts of cases which came under his own care. Monro accepted that cases of genuine smallpox could occur after successful vaccination but agreed that the cases were usually mild (Monro, 1818, pp. 145–208). However, some cases were still passed off as chickenpox, and some workers thought that a separate entity termed *varioloid* was the result. John Thomson published an account of 72 cases of the 'Varioloid Disease' which occurred in Edinburgh (Thomson, 1818). Of the 72 patients, 8 had already had smallpox in the past and 4 of these had very severe varioloid. Twenty-nine had been vaccinated in the past and only three of those had severe varioloid. Thirty-five of the patients had not had smallpox or been vaccinated and 9 of those patients died and another 13 had more or less severe varioloid. Six of these 35 patients developed varioloid after being inoculated with material from another patient. Thomson originally thought that the outbreak was one of chickenpox but abandoned that idea because of the severity. He thought that the disease in previously vaccinated patients was relatively mild, that it tended to have a 'varicelloid' disposition in infants, and that it showed 'more of the character of small-pox' in adults. So it seems clear that the varioloid disease in previously vaccinated individuals was smallpox which could transmit smallpox to contacts.

Perhaps Jenner's most serious error in the whole vaccination story was his failure to grasp the significance of attacks of smallpox in people who had been vaccinated. How close he got to it can perhaps be seen in a letter which he wrote to Evans of Ketley in 1805.

> The security given to the constitution by the vaccine inoculation is exactly equal to that given by the variolous. To expect more from it would be wrong. As failures in the latter are constantly presenting themselves . . . we must expect to find them in the former also (Baron, 1838, II, p. 29).

However, although Jenner conceded in private that cases of

smallpox would occasionally occur in the vaccinated, he was still reluctant to grasp the significance in public. In 1804 he published a short paper in the *Medical and Physical Journal* in which he discussed the failure of vaccination to take in those who had certain skin disorders, and recommended that such people should be revaccinated. However, he maintained that revaccination was not normally necessary in straightforward cases (Jenner, 1804). In 1821 he published a circular letter in which he emphasized that if smallpox occurred in someone who had been vaccinated, then the vaccination must have been faulty in some way (Jenner, 1821). Perhaps Jenner's last formal statements on vaccination were made in a letter written in July 1821 to Dr Gregory who had succeeded Woodville and Adams as physician to the Smallpox Hospital. In this letter, which was written for publication, Jenner stated that 'strict attention [to vaccination] as a general law will produce complete protection' and that 'varioloids in all their gradations' could occur if vaccination was done improperly (Gregory, 1822). So to the end Jenner firmly believed that correct vaccination would offer complete protection, although he admitted that variolation could not offer this degree of security. I suspect that he became increasingly convinced, partly through his own wishful thinking and partly through the influence of friends such as Baron, that his vaccination was very special in this respect.

The second answer to Creighton's conundrum about cowpox – when it produces morbid ulceration – also caused a lot of comment. However, a modern statement of what we must assume was Jenner's view is quite reasonable, i.e. sometimes genuine vaccines became contaminated with pathogenic bacteria and the resulting lesion produced an unacceptably severe reaction. In his discussion of the Stonehouse vaccinations, which as we have seen was thought by some to give severe reactions, Jenner wrote 'the most material indisposition, or at least that which is felt most sensibly, *does not arise primarily from the first action of the virus on the constitution, but that it often comes on, if the pustule is left to chance, as a secondary disease'* (Jenner, 1799, p. 32).

One famous incident in which vaccination produced unacceptably severe reactions occurred in late 1800 in Clapham, London. This incident was investigated in detail by Paytherus (1801, pp. 45–59). Some of the people concerned had been vaccinated on 22 October and some on 31 October with the same lancet which had not been cleaned in the intervening period. Initially the first series of vaccinations produced no untoward effects. However, when the lancet was used to

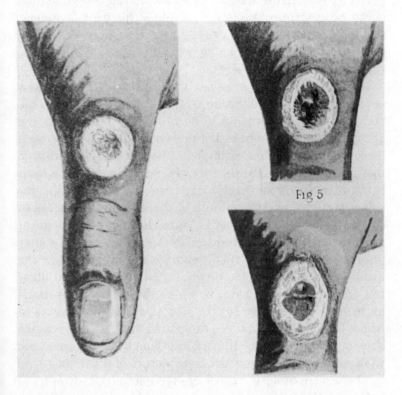

Figure 18 Accidental human cowpox. This shows some of the illustrations used by Crookshank to illustrate his original paper on cowpox in Wiltshire. This was written before his interest in Jenner and vaccination really started. (Author's Collection. Reproduced with the permission of the Editor of the *British Medical Journal*.)

take vaccine from J. Hall, one of the first series of patients, Hall then developed fatal erysipelas. Others who were vaccinated at the same time from other donors but with the same lancet had erysipelas to varying extent. Lettsom believed that the original vaccine, which he had also used, was satisfactory and concluded that 'the disease was not the cowpock but morbid ulceration, originating from the purulent matter formed under the scab, or dried pustule of the cowpock with which the patients were infected' (Lettsom, 1800). To this perfectly reasonable account of how bacterial contamination could be transmitted, Creighton added his own comment, 'Lettsom, whose writings prove him to have been something of a windbag, did not know what he was talking about' (Creighton, 1889, p. 179).

In some instances it is not possible to determine how severe the lesions really were. A good example of this is the contradictory accounts by Thornton and Hughes of the effects of the Stonehouse lymph which have already been discussed. As another example of how a person's attitude may affect the apparent severity of a particular lesion, we can again turn to Crookshank's experiences. To illustrate his sober, straightforward, account of the Wiltshire outbreak of cowpox (1888), he published coloured lithographs of some of the lesions; some are reproduced in Figure 18. When he later published his *History* (1889), and wished to emphasize the loathsomeness of cowpox, he published quite different illustrations of the same lesions in which the severity was much more apparent (Figure 19). In view of the circumstances in which Crookshank's *History* came to be written, it is reasonable to suppose that the illustrations which accompanied the 1888 paper gave the more accurate picture of the lesions.

There were other instances of severe lesions. However, as indicated above it is not always possible to determine just how severe they were. In addition, if they were severe it is not possible to determine with certainty whether this was an inherent property of the particular vaccine, or because the vaccine was contaminated with bacteria.

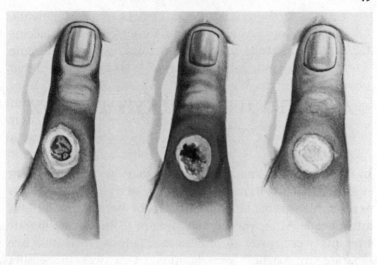

Figure 19 Accidental human cowpox. The same lesions as those shown in Figure 18, but redrawn by Crookshank for his *History* (1889). The left-hand lesion is the same in each case and 'Fig 5' (upper right) of Figure 18 corresponds to the central lesion in Figure 19. The increased severity of the redrawn lesions is obvious, even when reproduced in black-and-white. (Author's Collection.)

The problem of true and spurious cowpox, however much it may tell us about the effectiveness and acceptability of early vaccines, does not tell us anything about their origins. We can now take a look at post-Jennerian attempts to attenuate smallpox and see what is to be learnt from this.

11

Attenuation of Smallpox

In Chapter 3 I have suggested that there was no consistent evidence that smallpox virus was becoming so attenuated as to resemble vaccine virus in the years before vaccination was introduced. After vaccination became common deliberate attempts were made to attenuate smallpox virus and two separate approaches were adopted. One was the earlier method of arm-to-arm transfer in humans. However, now that vaccines were available for comparison the desired result was known. The second approach investigated the relationship between smallpox and cowpox by attempting to develop vaccine strains by growth of smallpox virus in animals, usually cows. Again vaccines were available for comparison and this was to cause a considerable amount of confusion.

Most accounts of attempts to produce vaccine by arm-to-arm transfer on the whole lacked detail. Curiously, Jenner was one of the first after the introduction of vaccination to consider the possibility of attenuating smallpox (1799, pp. 34–7). One of the first children he had vaccinated (Mary James) had been treated with caustic to destroy the virus only hours after it had been inoculated. Jenner later variolated this girl, she had a very mild response, and virus taken from her also produced a very mild response. Jenner believed that the original vaccination had brought about an attenuation of the smallpox virus, and suggested that it provided a method for producing a mild variety of smallpox.

One detailed account of attempts to attenuate smallpox was published by Joseph Adams in his *A Popular View of the Vaccine Inoculation* (1807). Adams, who succeeded Woodville as physician to the Smallpox Hospital, selected as his starting material a mild variety of smallpox which he called the 'pearl sort'. This may have been the same type which Jenner investigated in 1789 and which he called swinepox. In his *Popular View* Adams described the development of vaccine from pearl smallpox. The first person inoculated, William Croft, had a local lesion which resembled vaccine on the tenth day, but had about 150 pustules by the thirteenth day (Adams, 1807, pp. 28–9). Virus from Croft was used to inoculate Rogers whose local lesion 'was perfectly vaccine in all its stages' (*ibid.* p. 29). Mary Dobins was also inoculated with virus from Croft but no lesion developed. Dobins and four others were then inoculated with virus from Rogers (*ibid.* pp. 29–31). Four of them had arms which Adams described as 'perfect vaccine' and Dobins had no eruption. The other four had generalized eruptions; Eleanor Watts had 500 pustules, Richard Jude had 150, Elizabeth Grey had 60, and Thomas Dyson had an unspecified small number of pustules. Elizabeth Grey's local lesion was 'regularly vaccine to the 8th day' but on the twelfth day it was 'somewhat ragged with elevations round the vesicle'.

Seven patients were then inoculated from Dobins (Adams, 1807, pp. 31–2). Five of these had no eruptions and had local lesions which were 'vaccine in all the stages, and in the appearance of the scab'. The sixth patient had a local lesion which resembled vaccine but developed 100 pustules which appeared on the twelfth day. The seventh patient had a 'vaccine arm somewhat irregular, with fever, but with no pustules'. After one more arm-to-arm transfer Adams had to abandon this particular series because the parents of his patients had been influenced by 'enemies to vaccination', and were afraid that Adams had been using cowpox instead of the mild smallpox. However, in an appendix Adams described another series of smallpox inoculations 'approaching nearer to vaccination than any hitherto recorded' (*ibid.* pp. 153–8). He started with a patient who had been variolated because she had been exposed to natural smallpox. In all, 85 patients were inoculated from her and of these 64 had a 'circum-scribed vesicle resembling cowpox'. Of those of the 64 who were followed up only 8 had no generalized eruptions and 52 had generalized eruptions which appeared from the tenth to the seventeenth day. The first passage was made from a patient with no eruption and the recipients had no eruptions. A second passage was made to three subjects who had no eruptions. In later passages some patients had eruptions, and material from the secondary pustules caused smallpox for three passages.

There is in Adams's results an overall similarity to those of Woodville, and to Kelson's experience with Pearson's thread. It is possible that Adams did achieve attenuation, but if so it does not prove that this happened in Woodville's practice, merely that it could have. Again we have to consider the possibility of contamination, this time with vaccine. The difference between pre-Jennerian attempts to attenuate smallpox and the attempts made in the nineteenth century is that the later workers knew what they were looking for. Despite Jenner's initial ambiguity the differences between the local lesions of vaccine and inoculated smallpox were soon appreciated and were discussed and illustrated by many investigators (*see*, for example, Figure 10, p. 81). Adams was specifically looking for and selecting from lesions which most resembled the vaccines which had been introduced. If in these circumstances he had inadvertently got his smallpox material contaminated with genuine vaccine he would very soon have selected out the vaccine as explained in Chapter 8. Vaccines were being used extensively and the possibility of contamination must have been high.

Further attempts to attenuate smallpox in humans were reported from Europe but few details were given. For example Guillou, a French naval surgeon (referred to as Guillon by some), described some results obtained in December 1826 and January 1827 (Guillou, 1827). He used virus from a case of varioloid and apparently obtained typical vaccine vesicles in the first patient on which it was used.

Virus from this patient was used to inoculate 42 children and from these 100 patients were inoculated. Although it was stressed that the trials were carried out under close supervision, the lack of detail in Guillou's account makes any assessment impossible.

In 1839 Basil Thiele, the medical inspector for the Kazan district of Russia, published an account of his novel method of transforming smallpox into vaccinia and the important points have been translated by Razzell (1977a, pp. 93–4). Thiele stored smallpox virus between pieces of glass which were then sealed with wax and stored for ten days. The virus was then diluted with milk and inoculated into patients. Initially large vesicles were produced with two separate bouts of fever. By passing from arm to arm and continuing to dilute the virus with milk, Thiele found that the lesion started to resemble that produced by vaccine, and that only one bout of fever occurred. He recommended that ten serial transfers should be made but found that the vaccine character sometimes developed by about the fifth transfer. If the milk was omitted after only two or three subcultures the inoculated virus often caused smallpox. Without more details of the conditions in which he was working it is difficult to analyse Thiele's results.

With vaccination an established practice, variolation fell into disrepute and was gradually made illegal in most Western countries. It was, however, resorted to in emergencies when smallpox epidemics occurred and vaccine was in short supply. It was in these circumstances that Armand Trousseau the famous French clinician made his observations on variolation. He found, in the nineteenth century, the variability which is my impression of eighteenth century variolation also, and his comments speak for themselves.

> We obtained the desired result in some children to the extent that the mother pustule . . . was alone developed . . . This localized variola, without general eruption or serious symptoms, would perhaps be no more contagious than the

cow-pock. Unfortunately, matters did not turn out so propitiously. In some cases, I attained the complete success of having the pustule of inoculation; but in others, in which the very same virus had been employed, there were general eruptions, and worse still, communication of smallpox to the non-inoculated persons (Trousseau, 1869, pp. 92–3).

At the same time that these attempts were being made to develop vaccines from smallpox by arm-to-arm transfer, attempts were also made to infect animals, particularly cows, with smallpox virus. These attempts were made in part to investigate the relationship between cowpox and smallpox, and in part to try to establish new strains of vaccine.

In general the results obtained fell into one of three categories: those in which smallpox virus was apparently adapted to growth in the cow and became transformed into vaccinia; those in which limited growth of smallpox virus occurred but where no transformation took place; and those in which no adaptation or transformation took place. It should be noted that when attempts were successful they often formed a small minority of the total attempts.

There is not enough space here to discuss all these trials. They have been discussed before, by Crookshank and Creighton for example, and a little more objectively by S. A. Monckton Copeman in his Milroy lectures (1899). Unfortunately Copeman gave very few references but some are to be found in the reviews by Horgan (1938), and Herrlich and his colleagues (1963).

According to Copeman the first attempt to grow smallpox in cows was made by Gassner of Gunburg in 1807, who apparently infected a cow after ten unsuccessful attempts (Copeman, 1899, p. 42). However, Viborg, a Dane, successfully infected monkeys in 1792 although he failed to infect other animal species (Viborg, 1802). Thiele in addition to developing 'lacto-vaccine' in the way described above also reported in the same paper that he had twice produced vaccine by the inoculation of smallpox virus into cows. At about the same time more detailed reports were published independently by English workers. Robert Ceely, surgeon to the Buckinghamshire Infirmary, whose views on true and spurious cowpox were discussed in the previous chapter, also tried to infect cows with smallpox virus (Ceely, 1840). His initial attempts to infect cows by covering their heads with infected bedding failed; apparently this method had previously been used by Sonderland (Ceely, 1840, pp. 379–82). However, Ceely apparently succeeded in infecting two of the three calves he variolated in February 1839, although these successes were obtained in rather suspicious circumstances (Ceely, 1840, pp. 382–8). The first animal was inoculated with fourteen 'points' (actually the teeth from a comb) on one side of the vulva. The initial inflammation started to subside from the seventh day onward, but at one site a large lesion developed very quickly from the ninth to the tenth day after inoculation. The previous day Ceely had inoculated the animal in eleven places on the opposite side of the vulva with ordinary vaccine and the lesions at these sites developed as expected. Material taken from the smallpox lesion on the tenth day was used to 'vaccinate' five children with a total of twenty insertions of which only six took. None of the patients had a pustular eruption although one had a non-specific rash (pp. 403–5). Six out of twenty is a very low take rate for material from a fresh lesion the size of the one produced if the lesion was solely due to virus replication. It is possible that the lesion was just a large blister which became contaminated with vaccine either inadvertently by Ceely, or by the animal moving its tail. Ceely's second animal was inoculated with smallpox in the same way and at the same time as the first and the lesions again started to regress. On the fourteenth day the animal was re-inoculated with smallpox at eight sites and six days later they all showed a typical vaccine appearance. The day before this re-inoculation Ceely had charged some points from the genuine vaccination sites on the first animal. Again transfer of the smallpox material to children gave typical vaccine reactions with no general eruptions and the vaccine established apparently from smallpox virus in these experiments was widely used (pp. 406–21).

The conclusion of many people who have analysed Ceely's results was that the smallpox inoculation sites became contaminated with vaccine in some way. Certainly he was using vaccine at the same time and using a great number of points. In addition to the use of vaccine mentioned above Ceely also vaccinated a fourth calf at the same time that he initially variolated the other three (*Report*, 1840, p. 10).

At the same time that Ceely was starting his investigations John Badcock, a Brighton chemist, was starting his own series of extensive investigations, some of which were summarized in a small pamphlet published in 1845 and reprinted by Crookshank (1889, II, pp. 513–27). Unfortunately Badcock gives very few details. Material taken from the cow three days after variolation was used on his son and produced a vaccine take. Badcock mentioned 'other occasionally successful cases' occurring in experiments on 'upwards of ninety cows'. Much later Copeman wrote that during a period of 25 years Badcock repeated the experiment more than 500 times and was successful on 38 occasions; unfortunately it is not clear where Copeman obtained this information. According to Winterburn (1886), who also gave no references, similar results were obtained in America by Adams and Putnam in 1849, and by Van Bibber and Knight in 1852.

Even at the end of the nineteenth century, when the need to avoid contamination was better appreciated, the experiments that were made are open to some criticism. Many were carried out in vaccine institutes or used vaccine as a control. In some cases the cows were taken to the smallpox wards and inoculated there from the patients. It can be reasonably assumed that where there was smallpox there would also be vaccine and it must have been extremely difficult to ensure that the suspensions of smallpox virus used had not become contaminated. Monckton Copeman, whose own experiments will be discussed below, 'confessed, that seeing the conditions under which they were carried out, many, particularly of the earlier experiments are of little worth' (Copeman, 1899, p. 62).

The type of experiment Copeman had in mind was that described by Thomas Whiteside Hime of the Bradford Vaccine Establishment in 1892. Although Hime considered that 'there is no weak spot in the chain of evidence' there are enough weak spots in his experiment to raise a reasonable doubt about his conclusions. He was working in a vaccine establishment and inoculated his calf on 'the ordinary vaccine table'; this could have been the source of contamination, if this is the explanation of Hime's results. The shaved skin of the calf was then inoculated with smallpox virus. The skin, with the inevitable small scratches, would have been very sensitive and it is perhaps most significant that three of the four lesions which developed were 'at places quite distinct from any insertions'. Those who came to inspect Hime's calf were struck by the 'specific pock-like appearance' of the lesions. It is not unreasonable to suggest that Hime's results were caused by contamination with vaccine.

Copeman carried out his own experiments in which he believed that the possibility of contamination had been eliminated, as he was working at the Brown Institute in which vaccine had not previously been used. These experiments formed the basis for his belief that smallpox and cowpox (i.e. vaccine) were not independent but that cowpox was a stable variant of smallpox. In his first series of experiments he attempted to grow smallpox in cows and was apparently successful on one out of four attempts. On the first passage in the calf, smallpox produced only a superficial inflammation and only a very slight tendency to vesiculate. Material from this first animal produced more marked lesions in a second calf, and by the third transfer Copeman considered the results to be quite unequivocal (Copeman, 1899, pp. 58–60). However, four subsequent attempts to repeat this experiment failed (Copeman, 1903). His colleague Dr E. Klein apparently succeeded in some instances but his experiments were carried out at the Government Vaccine Establishment (Klein, 1894).

Copeman apparently achieved consistent success in producing vaccine in calves by inoculating them with material taken from variolated monkeys. However, in this case, although the monkeys had been infected in the Brown Institute, the calves were infected in the Government Vaccine Establishment. Smallpox virus will grow well in monkeys and there is no reason to criticize the first part of the experiment. However, it is possible that in the second part the calves also became infected with vaccine, particularly since all the animals responded promptly. There is also another explanation which has not previously been considered. Monkeys are susceptible to infection with monkeypox virus, and outbreaks of monkeypox have been reported in captive animals in research establishments (Arita and Henderson, 1968). Of particular significance is the fact that monkeypox virus can remain latent in the monkey and then be stimulated to produce infection when the animal is subjected to trauma (McConnell et al., 1962). It is possible that in Copeman's experiments the smallpox infection provided this trauma, and that the calves were then inoculated with a mixture of smallpox and monkeypox viruses. Monkeypox has a much wider host range than smallpox virus and would be expected to grow in calves. In 1938 E. S. Horgan of Khartoum reported successful results very similar to those of Copeman. Horgan believed he had eliminated the possibility of contamination with vaccine.

The prompt and general success of Copeman's monkey experiments contrasts strongly with his one success in eight calf experiments in which smallpox became slowly and poorly adapted. That this success in calves was an isolated one and the adaptation was gradual suggests that it might have been a genuinely successful result. However, before we accept it we should remember that the criteria by which vaccinia and smallpox were differentiated were few, and that as discussed earlier (Chapter 8, pp. 111–12) the transformation of smallpox into vaccinia would involve important alterations in the genetic structure of the virus. Consequently it is possible that what Copeman, Horgan, and others who obtained similar results achieved was not transformation but rather an attenuation and adaptation of smallpox virus.

Although concern was expressed about the possibility of contamination with vaccine both Copeman and the Royal Commissioners considered that so many attempts had been made that some successes must have been genuine. This view was generally accepted in Britain and Germany for the first thirty or so years of the twentieth century. The view of the British 'Establishment' was presented by F. R. Blaxall of the Ministry of Health who wrote the chapter on smallpox in *A System of Bacteriology* published in 1930 by the Medical Research Council:

> Beside the monkey, variola can be inoculated on many other animals . . . but once vesiculation is produced and perhaps carried on for one or two removes the disease apparently ceases to be variola . . . in fact, it has become vaccinia . . . probably all animals susceptible to vaccinia are inoculable with variola (Blaxall, 1930, pp. 104–5).

A similar view was the official German position (Gins, 1938). This opinion was consistently challenged by French workers, however. Experiments on the subject were commissioned by the Society of Medical Sciences of Lyons which appointed Dr A. Chauveau to supervise the trials and prepare a report. This he did in 1865 and a concise summary in English was provided by the Royal Commissioners. Briefly Chauveau and his colleagues found that inoculation of human smallpox material into cows did not produce a vaccine lesion. Instead there was thickening and inflammation which if punctured developed into a papule. Inoculation of material squeezed from such a papule produced the same effect when inoculated into a second cow. On occasions a third transfer could be made but never a fourth. That no transformation or even attenuation had occurred was demonstrated by the fact that 'veritable smallpox' was produced in human subjects inoculated with the bovine material (Royal Commission, 1898, pp. 201–2). According to Crookshank and Copeman, neither of whom gave references, a Dr Martin of Boston, Mass. obtained a similar result in 1860 (1836 according to Crookshank), when he inoculated 50 people with material from a cow which had been variolated. Nearly all the people developed smallpox and three died (Copeman, 1899, p. 49).

Chauveau maintained his interest in the subject for many years, and did more experiments in cows, calves, and horses. In 1891 in a long two-part paper in which he discussed the problem he succinctly and emphatically summarized the results of nearly thirty years work:

> *En un mot, le virus vaccinal n'est pas du virus variolique atténué* (Chauveau, 1891, p. 566).

Another French group which challenged the English and German view was led by L. F. A. Kelsch and P. Teissier who investigated the problem for over twenty years. In 1909 and 1910 they reported the failure of twenty attempts to transform smallpox virus. In particular they also provided dramatic evidence of the ease with which contamination with vaccine could occur. Calves which had been shaved and scarified in a vaccine laboratory and then inoculated with sterile glycerol developed vaccine lesions caused by virus which must have been circulating in the atmosphere (Kelsch et al., 1909, 1910). Glycerol, which kills contaminating bacteria and enables vaccine to be stored in liquid suspension at $-20°C$, was generally used as a suspending medium for vaccine. Its use was discontinued in Britain in 1979. Later Teissier showed that monkeys could be infected with smallpox but that the virus obtained from the monkeys would not infect calves or rabbits (Teissier et al., 1911), and in 1931 reported more failures this time using intratesticular inoculation of virus from variolated monkeys into young bulls, dogs, and donkeys (Teissier et al., 1931).

More recent attempts to investigate the problem have

confirmed the views of the French workers and failed to confirm the early English and German views. The most extensive attempts were made over a number of years in Germany by Professor A. Herrlich and his colleagues (1963). These experiments were made in the full knowledge of the need to exclude vaccinia and to characterize properly any virus isolated from the variolated animals. The experiments were carried out in premises either newly-built or rebuilt specially for the studies. Herrlich's efficiency in excluding vaccinia can be judged from his simple conclusion:

All experiments failed to produce transformation of variola- or alastrim virus into vaccinia virus.

The results obtained were divided into two groups, one consisting of hosts in which smallpox virus would grow easily and one consisting of hosts in which little or no growth took place. In fact apart from man, the only animal in the accepted sense of the word in which smallpox will grow readily is the monkey. It can be grown in the brain of suckling mice and in the fertile chick embryo but these methods, like the use of cell cultures, should be regarded as rather artificial techniques available only to virologists. Although Herrlich and his colleagues infected monkeys they found no evidence that the virus was becoming transformed into vaccinia. They tried other hosts in which little or no reaction occurred including rabbits, pigs, sheep, goats, and calves. In some cases they noticed a slight local reaction but were either unable to recover virus at all from the lesions or did not recover enough to be able to infect a second animal. Significantly Herrlich's group failed in three particular respects to confirm earlier claims. Firstly they failed to infect calves directly as had Ceely, Badcock, Hime, etc. Secondly they failed to infect calves indirectly with material from variolated monkeys as had Copeman. Thirdly they failed to transfer monkey-adapted smallpox virus to rabbits as Horgan had done. Herrlich's work has had considerable influence on those modern virologists who believe that vaccinia is not derived from smallpox virus.

I have already described (Chapter 8, p. 112) how Dumbell and Bedson succeeded with difficulty in adapting smallpox virus to growth in the rabbit skin. This result should not be regarded as a refutation of Herrlich since they carefully adapted the virus to grow in rabbit cell cultures first before proceeding to adapt that virus to the rabbit skin. Like Herrlich they took particular care to prevent contamination with vaccinia virus, and although the lesions which the adapted smallpox virus produced in the rabbit looked like those produced by vaccinia, the rabbit-adapted virus behaved like smallpox virus in all other respects tested.

In summary, when we try to evaluate the attempts of the early workers we have to bear in mind five important points. Firstly, the extremely limited host range of smallpox virus which has been shown by properly conducted up-to-date experiments. Secondly, that sufficient care was not always taken to exclude contamination with vaccine which was often used as a control. Thirdly, the fact that vaccine (and cowpox) has a wider host range than smallpox virus and will out-grow it under virtually all circumstances. Fourthly, that the methods used by the early workers would not differentiate adequately between, say, calf-adapted smallpox and vaccine, Fifthly, that transformation of smallpox to vaccinia would require radical and major changes in the genetic structure of the virus, in effect the production of a new type of virus, and this is most unlikely to occur.

The post-Jennerian attempts to attenuate smallpox by arm-to-arm transfer in humans were poorly controlled and inadequately described. They add nothing more to the solution of the problem concerning the origins of vaccinia than the results of the pre-Jennerian variolators which have been described in Chapter 3, and I have argued in Chapters 8 and 9 that smallpox was unlikely to be involved in the origin of the Woodville/Pearson vaccines except possibly as one parent of a hybrid.

The validity of the many claims to have derived vaccine by variolation of animals is inevitably compromised by the possibility that contamination with vaccine occurred. Many of the workers were aware of this problem and took such precautions as they thought fit, though due to the low level of microbiological knowledge existing at the time, those precautions were often unsatisfactory by modern standards. Contamination with vaccine almost certainly occurred on many occasions but this does not necessarily mean that it happened in all cases. The experiments in which contamination was most likely to have occurred are those where there was an immediate and dramatic result such as in the detailed accounts of Ceely and Hime. Where the effect was slight and gradual as in some of the experiments of Copeman and Klein it is possible that an adaptation occurred similar to that achieved by Dumbell and Bedson. However, if this was the case then the product would have been a host range variant of smallpox rather than what would now be recognized as vaccinia. If vaccinia was to have been produced in this way then such a host range mutant would have to be the important first step to enable the other necessary mutants to be selected out, giving a slow, gradual transformation.

Crookshank was one person who did not believe that any contamination had occurred, and he considered most emphatically that there had been no transformation of smallpox virus into vaccinia. He believed that the vaccines which had been developed from variolated cows by such as Ceely and Badcock were still smallpox. 'I repeat', he wrote, 'that all those who have been inoculated with Ceely's or Badcock's "variola-vaccine" lymph have not, in the true sense of the word, been *vaccinated; they have not been Cow Poxed, but they have been variolated*' (Crookshank, 1889, 1, p. 301).

It is just possible that a very small proportion of the mid or late nineteenth-century vaccines may have been derived from smallpox virus, although reasons for doubting that they have survived into the twentieth century will be discussed in Chapter 13. Some writers have tended to assume that there was just one origin for vaccinia, but to accept that some vaccines may have been derived from smallpox should not weaken an argument that proposes that the majority were derived from some other source. However, I believe that in order to determine the origin of the majority of the vaccine strains we have to examine poxviruses other than smallpox that were available to the early vaccinators.

12

Cowpox and Grease

In previous chapters the terms *cowpox*, *vaccine*, and *vaccinia* have been used more or less interchangeably. This was unavoidable because until 1939 it was not known that vaccinia and cowpox viruses were distinct and consequently it is not possible to determine with certainty which virus was being used by earlier workers. Such limited circumstantial evidence as is available will be discussed in the next chapter. Blaxall in his chapter on Animal Pock Diseases in the MRC *System of Bacteriology* gave the terms 'variolae vaccinae; vaccinia; vaccine', as synonyms for cowpox (Blaxall, 1930, p. 150). In fact as recently as 1963 some American writers considered that cowpox and vaccinia were synonymous (Williams, 1963, pp. 14–15). However, the two viruses were shown to be clearly different in 1939 by Allan W. Downie and all later work on the subject has confirmed the differences between them. The nature and significance of these differences will be discussed in the next chapter. Before 1939 those interested in the origins of vaccinia had basically to decide whether vaccinia was the natural disease of cows (i.e. cowpox) or whether it might be derived from smallpox as discussed in the last chapter. After 1939 they had to account for the fact that cowpox and vaccinia were distinct. This has two important consequences. Firstly, because vaccinia is not now found naturally in the field, it has been assumed or argued that it never occurred naturally and so must have been derived from viruses which did occur naturally then. Secondly, because vaccinia is distinct from cowpox, those who believe it is not derived from smallpox have had to consider how it could have been derived from cowpox. This as we will presently see presents problems almost as great as those involved in considering an origin from smallpox. Three assumptions have usually been made, and these are not necessarily justified. One is that because vaccinia is not found now it must never have occurred naturally. Another is that cowpox was ever enzootic in cows. The third is that what the early vaccinators referred to as cowpox was caused by a virus which we would now recognize as cowpox. When discussing the origins of vaccinia previous writers have given too little attention to the possibility that poxviruses other than smallpox and cowpox may have been circulating in Europe during the early nineteenth century. If other viruses did exist they provide another possible origin for vaccinia. The obvious candidate is horsepox – Jenner's grease. Before discussing the possibility that other poxviruses were present it might be appropriate to say something about cowpox itself, because there has always been something of a mystery about it and recent work has to some extent added to the mystery.

Cowpox virus was so named because the first strain to be characterized was isolated from a farmworker who had been infected whilst handling infected cattle. Since then the virus has been isolated on a number of occasions over the years, either from farmworkers who had been in contact with infected cattle, or from the cattle themselves. Bovine cowpox is a relatively trivial infection and outbreaks are usually reported only when human cases occur or when many cattle are involved. However, human infection is relatively severe and about half of the patients are admitted to hospital. Consequently medical aid will be sought when human infection occurs and few if any human cases will go unreported. Although cattle undoubtedly do get infected and transmit the infection to man, recent evidence has failed to confirm the assumption that the cow is the natural reservoir of the virus named after it. Until recently it has been assumed that cowpox is enzootic in cattle, but a comparison of cowpox outbreaks with infections such as pseudocowpox which is known to be enzootic in cattle shows many striking differences. Pseudocowpox has been recognized in many herds and in a survey in Southwest England about 13 per cent of animals inspected in abattoirs were found to be infected (Gibbs and Osborne, 1974). Human infection with pseudo-cowpox virus occurs in farmworkers and abattoir workers and such human infections can be traced back to cattle. The incidence of human infection varies from year to year. It is a relatively painless infection in man and not all cases may seek medical help, but about 30 to 50 cases per year are reported to the Public Health Laboratory Service in England and Wales. The contrast with cowpox is quite marked. Despite the greater severity of human cowpox only one or two cases per year are reported in England and Wales. This low incidence means that surveys to obtain meaningful information must be carried out for some years and I have reviewed the situation in England and Wales from 1965 to 1976 (Baxby, 1977a). During this period there were only twelve outbreaks in all, and of these two involved cattle only. In only three of the ten human cases were cattle involved. All the cases occurred in different geographical areas at different times and there was no connection between any of them. Seven human cases were particularly interesting because detailed inquiries failed to establish direct contact with infected cattle, although all the patients lived in, or had visited, rural areas. Most significant was the failure to detect any general evidence of cowpox in cattle. Although infected cattle were involved in three of the human outbreaks we were unable to determine how the herds became infected, no further outbreaks developed from them, and cowpox was not detected in neighbouring herds. Detailed inquiries also failed to detect any evidence of recent bovine cowpox in the localities where the seven human cases which were unconnected with cattle had occurred. In addition to looking for clinically ill cattle a survey was made of serum samples from over 1,000 cows from the localities in which the human cases occurred but no antibodies to cowpox were detected. If cowpox was enzootic in cattle we would expect it to occur in cattle with an incidence similar to that of pseudocowpox, would expect more human cases to occur, and would expect most if not all the human cases to be traceable to cattle. This is not the case. The current view is that cows are not the natural reservoir of 'cowpox' virus, that both cows and humans become infected accidentally, and that the actual reservoir is some as yet unknown animal, probably a small wild mammal. So far attempts to identify the reservoir have failed. In 1977 and 1978 cowpox was recognized in cheetahs in two English zoos where it infected five valuable animals and killed four of them (Baxby *et al.*, 1979). Obviously the cheetahs became infected accidentally and again detailed inquiries failed to detect cowpox in the local cattle or to trace the source. A similar situation exists in Europe where viruses related to cowpox occasionally cause serious infections in zoo and circus animals (Baxby, 1977b).

Because 'true' cowpox infection in cows is now so rare, and most of the bovine teat infections are caused by what Jenner would recognize as spurious cowpox, i.e. pseudocowpox, bovine herpes mammillitis, and warts, we must consider whether cowpox ever was enzootic in cattle during the eighteenth and nineteenth centuries. This is not an easy question to answer because much of the available evidence is circumstantial. We know that Jenner was correct in his assertion that there were different types of bovine teat disease and that only one protected against smallpox, but we know nothing about the relative incidence of cowpox and the other infections during this period. However, the fact that there were many more reports of spurious cowpox than of true cowpox in the years immediately following the introduction of vaccination probably indicates that true cowpox was relatively uncommon. As mentioned previously, differential clinical diagnosis is not easy and the only bovine infections described in the early literature which we can accept as being due to cowpox are those in which the immunity of the animal or human patient was tested by subsequent vaccination or variolation, and very few such accounts are available. Due to the difficulties of making a differential diagnosis on the sick animal it is probable that the designation of true or spurious was made, not on the basis of the appearance of the lesions on the cow, but retrospectively on the results obtained when the virus was used as vaccine.

It is clear that even Jenner, who was particularly interested in the problem and who was working in a dairy county, had difficulty in obtaining supplies of cowpox. The most obvious evidence of this is the fact that after vaccinating Phipps in May 1796 he was unable to obtain more virus until March 1798. And after that he had to rely on the virus from London supplied by Woodville in 1799. One difficulty is caused by Jenner's tendency to give insufficient detail of his unsuccessful attempts. For example, in his *Further Observations* he wrote, 'I have often been foiled in my efforts to communicate the Cow Pox by inoculation' but did not give any further details (1799, p. 39). Consequently it is not possible to determine whether he was using material from old cowpox lesions or whether he was using material from a case of say, bovine herpes mammillitis.

Ceely's work has been mentioned before. He provided one of the best and most detailed descriptions of all aspects of cowpox, and his opinion on its incidence is worth quoting.

> The disease is occasionally epizootic . . . more commonly sporadic or nearly solitary. It may be seen sometimes at several contiguous farms, at other times one or two farms . . . entirely escape its visitation. Many years may elapse before it recurs at a given farm or vicinity, although all the animals may have been changed in the meantime' (Ceely, 1840, pp. 298–9).

That Ceely was investigating true cowpox was shown by the fact that effective vaccines were introduced from the viruses isolated.

The next outbreak of true cowpox to be reported in England was the one investigated by Crookshank in 1888, although there must have been unreported outbreaks in the intervening period. In his *History* Crookshank gave detailed accounts of outbreaks of cowpox in France, at Passy near Paris in 1836, at Eysine in Bordeaux in 1881 and 1884, and at Cérons in 1884, from which vaccines were established

(Crookshank, 1889, II, pp. 311–22). Crookshank tried to obtain evidence on the incidence of cowpox in the nineteenth century and concluded that it was relatively common. However, apart from the exception of certain parts of Germany, Crookshank's data in fact show that cowpox was probably as rare then as it is now, with outbreaks occurring relatively infrequently (Crookshank, 1889, I, pp. 454–8). Consequently there must be serious doubt about whether cowpox really was enzootic in the nineteenth century.

A term which has often been used in association with cowpox is *spontaneous*. Originally Jenner regarded spontaneous cowpox as spurious, but later, as already explained, he recognized some types of spontaneous cowpox as having protective effect against smallpox. Later in the nineteenth century investigators tried to take account of the supposed relationships between vaccine (i.e. cowpox), smallpox, and horsepox. Consequently the term 'spontaneous cowpox' was used if those investigating an outbreak suspected that there was no possibility of it having originated from a case of smallpox, horsepox or from a recently vaccinated individual. For instance Ceely wrote, 'For many years past, however, the spontaneous origin of the variolae vaccinae in the cow has not been doubted here' (Ceely, 1840, p. 299). On the other hand, Monckton Copeman investigated an outbreak of cowpox and could not trace the source. Believing as he did that vaccine (i.e. cowpox) could be produced from smallpox, he regarded as significant the fact that some of the cattle had been recently bought from an area which was having a smallpox epidemic (Copeman, 1904).

I have suggested in the last chapter that it is extremely unlikely that smallpox virus was transformed into vaccinia in the cow under experimental conditions, and so it is even more unlikely that it would have occurred naturally. Essentially the decision that an outbreak was one of spontaneous cowpox would have been made on epidemiological grounds.

The fact that many outbreaks of cowpox in the nineteenth century proved to have no known source and were referred to as spontaneous could be interpreted as indicating that the infection was being transmitted to cows from an unknown reservoir as is believed to happen at present.

Jenner was criticized for giving such a brief description of bovine cowpox and for not providing an illustration of it. Perhaps the first illustration of bovine cowpox to be published was that of Sacco and a copy of it accompanied the English review of his *Osservazioni* (Sacco, 1802). This engraving is generally regarded as a misrepresentation for what Sacco did was to depict on an illustration of the bovine udder, the progress of a typical smallpox lesion as it would appear on human skin. In fact both natural observations and experimental inoculation of cows with cowpox and vaccinia viruses show that the lesions produced in the cow by these viruses do not go through the same orderly progression as does the human smallpox lesion (Lauder *et al.*, 1971, Gibbs *et al.*, 1973). In particular the vesicular and pustular stage is absent and the bovine lesions progress from a papule to an ulcerated sore which then scabs. Figure 17, which has already been described (*see* p. 139), shows a scabbed lesion of cowpox, and Figure 20 shows more clearly the ulcerated lesions at an earlier stage in a different animal. At this stage vaccinia and cowpox in the human would be producing a vesicle. Ceely illustrated his account of cowpox and one of his plates, which is reproduced in Figure 21, shows a group of lesions in various stages of development. The illustration included by Crookshank in his 1888 paper is not very informative, showing as it does only old scabbed lesions. The illustration in his *History* (Crookshank, 1889, I, plate X) was chosen to show 'phagedaenic ulceration' and to fit his later views that cowpox was a severe disease. Even so the case depicted by Crookshank is not particularly severe when compared with those shown in Figures 17 and 20.

We can now examine Jenner's grease theory. I have mentioned how he initially believed that his vaccine originated in a disease of horses called *grease*, how he then tacitly accepted that vaccines derived from spontaneous cowpox were genuine, and how he dropped any formal reference to

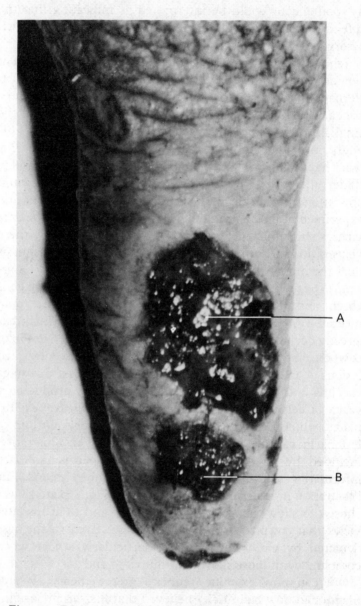

Figure 20 Bovine cowpox, 1970. A = ulcerated lesion, B = scabbed lesion. From Gibbs *et al.*, (1970, 1973). (Reproduced with the permission of Dr Gibbs and the Editor of the *Veterinary Record*.)

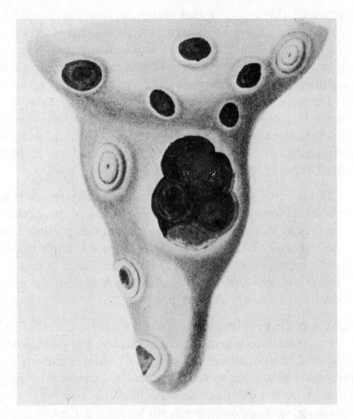

Figure 21 Bovine cowpox, 1840. Plate 2 Fig. 1 from Ceely's paper showing lesions in various stages of development. (Liverpool Medical Institution.)

the grease theory after 1799. There was no mention of it at all in his third pamphlet *A Continuation of Facts* (1800) nor in his fourth *The Origin of the Vaccine Inoculation* published in 1801. The omission of any mention of grease from this last pamphlet is perhaps the most significant because the *Origin* was intended to be a short, more or less popular, account of Jenner's work on vaccination up to that time.

Much circumstantial evidence was published on the subject, for example in Pearson's *Inquiry* and in the *Medical and Physical Journal*, and most of it was critical of Jenner's idea. The probable reason why Jenner dropped the grease theory was partly this criticism and partly the fact that all attempts to prove the theory by experiment had failed. However, as with most of Jenner's ideas there was some truth in the grease theory. The problem was in many ways similar to the confusion over true and spurious cowpox, and was aggravated by Jenner's unfortunate choice of the term grease. Even Baron, Jenner's friend and biographer, was confused by this. In 1838, twenty-five years after Jenner's death, and after completing his two-volume biography of Jenner, Baron added a short note.

> I take this opportunity of expressing my regret that I have employed the word *grease* in alluding to the disease in the horse. *Variolae equinae* is the proper designation. It has no necessary connexion with the grease though the disorders frequently co-exist. This circumstance at first misled Dr Jenner and it has caused much apprehension and confusion (Baron, 1838, II, p. 456).

This was the problem in a nutshell. Horses were subject to various infections one of which, horsepox, was immunologically related to smallpox and so would confer immunity to it. However, according to some critics the term grease should not have been applied to this particular infection.

Jenner had obtained virus from his friend Tanner in 1800 which was believed to have come from horses, but the first independent evidence in support of Jenner's view was published by Dr John Loy, a Yorkshire physician who was assisted by a surgeon with the same surname (Loy, 1801). Mr Loy obtained virus from the lesions on the hand of a man who had been treating horses suffering from what Loy referred to as grease. Virus from the man was used to inoculate his brother and the result was a lesion which 'had exactly the appearances of the genuine Cowpox' (Loy, 1801, pp. 8–10). However, Loy was not allowed to variolate the patient. Dr Loy also obtained virus from the original patient and inoculated a cow and a child with it. The child's lesion started to develop on the third day. By the sixth day there was dullish inflammation, by the eighth a vesicle, and by the fourteenth, a dark brown scab. The child resisted variolation (Loy, 1801, p. 13). The lesion in the cow started to develop on the fifth day and the 'inflammation, vesication, and scabbing were found to correspond so exactly with these appearances in mild cases of genuine Cowpox, that they admitted only of a similar description'. A child was inoculated with material from this cow but without any effect (*ibid*., p. 12). Loy also started a second series of experiments with material 'from a sore in the heel of a horse with the Grease'. This again was inoculated onto the teats of a cow, and material from the cow was used to inoculate a child who successfully resisted variolation (*ibid*., pp. 15–16). Virus from the horse was also used to inoculate a child directly and five children were inoculated from this child. All were variolated without effect (*ibid*., pp. 16–17).

So Loy had succeeded in demonstrating that there was an equine virus which was transmissible to cows, and that people inoculated with it resisted inoculated smallpox. However, Jenner believed that the horse virus had to pass through the cow before it was reliably effective in humans whereas Loy's experiments suggested that the horse virus was effective when transmitted directly to humans. Loy also pointed out a possible explanation for earlier failures to isolate horsepox virus – for this is what the horse virus can conveniently be called. Loy explained that he had failed on a number of occasions to transmit grease to both cows and humans. This led him to conclude that there were two kinds of grease, one of which, relatively rare was the horsepox (*ibid*., pp. 19–20). He noted that his successful attempts had been with virus taken from horses with a generalized infection whereas the unsuccessful attempts were made from animals with a localized infection.

Loy's results were brought to the attention of Jenner who regarded them as confirmation of his original theory. For example he sent a copy of Loy's pamphlet to the Duke of Clarence together with a letter in which he wrote that Loy's work 'decisively proves my early assertions'. He also wrote in a similar vein to de Carro who prepared French and German translations of Loy's pamphlet. However, despite these informal and personal acknowledgements of Loy's work Jenner never formally readopted the horsepox theory in his publications. Perhaps after originally having conceived the idea only to have it generally criticized, then having dropped all reference to it, Jenner was reluctant to draw public attention to it again. Particularly so since Loy's work did not prove Jenner's theory precisely, but suggested that the horse virus was effective on direct transfer to man.

More confirmation of the horsepox theory came from the Continent. Sacco described his discovery in a letter written to Jenner in March 1803 (Baron, 1838, 1, pp. 250–1). He recalled his earlier failures and explained how Loy's results had encouraged him to try further. Like Loy he had tried to inoculate cows as well as people and had obtained satisfactory results in people who had been inoculated directly with material from the horses. He suggested that vaccines could be derived from horses without the need for transfer through the cow and suggested that the virus could be called *equine* instead of vaccine. As in his earlier studies Sacco sent material to de Carro and this led to a minor confusion. Many years later in a letter to Alexander Monro, de Carro was to write that the virus which he had distributed so widely in the East (*see* Chapter 9) was Sacco's equine strain (Monro, 1826). However, de Carro was mistaken because the virus was sent to the East in 1801 and Sacco's equine strain was not introduced until 1803.

De Carro also wrote to tell Jenner of the discovery of horse-pox in Macedonia by Lafont, a French physician (Baron, 1838, 1, pp. 431–3). Again Loy's work had provided the stimulus. Lafont recognized the two different types of grease and used material from the type which the farriers referred to as 'variolous' and which, like Loy's, tended to produce a more generalized infection in the horses.

More equine strains were introduced in Britain and were used by Jenner but unfortunately no detailed accounts of their development were published. In 1813 Jenner wrote to Dr James Moore, Director of the National Vaccine Establishment and brother of Sir John Moore of Corunna, that he had obtained equine virus from a Mr Melon of Litchfield and had been 'using [it] from arm-to-arm for these two months past' (Baron, 1838, II, p. 386). In 1817 Jenner supplied the National Vaccine Establishment with another equine strain which according to Crookshank was very widely used (Crookshank, 1889, I, pp. 392–3).

Crookshank was unable to obtain any data on horsepox in Britain but visited France to obtain first-hand information about outbreaks which Peuch had investigated at Rieumes near Toulouse in 1880 and in Algeria in 1882. He also reviewed in detail an earlier outbreak at Rieumes in 1860 and an outbreak at Alfort in 1863 (Crookshank, 1889, I, pp. 395–418). These investigations confirmed the results of those workers who had investigated the problem at the beginning of the nineteenth century, and provided strains of vaccine which were widely used.

Horsepox was regarded as an independent equine disease which was transmissible to man where it produced a lesion similar to that produced by commercial vaccine or cowpox, and also induced immunity to these viruses. Other equine infections were also discussed and the guidelines for differential diagnosis were laid down. Of the three equine diseases described, horsepox produced the least specific picture, tending to cause a generalized eruption with lesions that were particularly noticeable around the mouth. However, the eruption did also occur on the legs, which might lead to the incorrect diagnosis of grease (*eaux aux jambes*). Lesions also tended to occur on the genital mucosa and the infection could be sexually transmitted, which might lead to the incorrect diagnosis of *maladie du coït*. The French workers encountered mixed infections which made diagnosis difficult but stressed the fact that the lesions of grease and *maladie du coït* were more localized and the infections were not transmissible to man.

Grease is still recognized, although the role of microorganisms in its production is not clear and environmental factors are believed to play a major role. It is found in horses which have been kept in wet and muddy conditions and their transfer to dry paddocks usually leads to recovery. It has been suggested that a fungus, *Dermatophilus congolensis*, may play some role (Hungerford, 1975, p. 760).

Unfortunately horsepox became extinct in the early years of the present century and no studies have been made on viruses from horsepox since reliable techniques for poxvirus identification were developed. The term horsepox is still used colloquially to refer to *equine coital exanthem*, an infection caused by a herpes virus and probably the same infection as the *maladie du coït* described by the nineteenth-century workers. Probably the last outbreak of genuine horsepox in England was the one investigated by Blaxall in 1901 and his brief account contains nothing of significance (Blaxall, 1903). Horsepox does not seem to have been a very common infection in the nineteenth century. It is possible that the true reservoir of the virus was not the horse and that, as with cowpox, some unknown small wild animal was involved.

The lack of virological information means that the recognition of horsepox as a clinical entity relied heavily on epidemiological studies which can be untrustworthy. Nevertheless it is clear that outbreaks of horsepox did occur in the nineteenth century and that vaccine strains were established from them. Horsepox should therefore be included in any discussion of the origins of vaccinia.

13

The Origins of Vaccinia

The mystery concerning the origins of smallpox vaccine is not just limited to the early nineteenth-century strains. It extends to all strains because those used today were introduced before adequate laboratory methods for virus characterization were available and also before regulations required the pedigree of a vaccine to be recorded. The supply and distribution of vaccine was under only loose control until the early twentieth century. Brief accounts of this topic have been published by Hutchinson (1947) and Dudgeon (1963).

The National Vaccine Establishment (NVE) was instituted in 1808. It developed from the moribund Royal Jennerian Institution and Jenner was initially appointed as Director. However, he soon resigned because he thought he was not given sufficient power, and was replaced by James Moore. The NVE was administered jointly by the Royal Colleges of Surgeons and Physicians until 1861 when it came under the control of the Privy Council. The NVE and other private concerns such as the Smallpox Hospital distributed vaccine throughout Britain, to the Army and Navy, and, if requested, abroad. The first Vaccination Act of 1840 made variolation illegal and legislated for the supply of vaccine. Until the 1880s the bulk of vaccine used in Britain was maintained by arm-to-arm transfer. This meant that well-organized vaccinators could operate independently of the official suppliers by obtaining material when those who had been vaccinated returned for examination. It also meant that the vaccine suppliers had to have susceptible vaccinees available in order to continue the line of vaccine.

Vaccine produced on the skin of calves (calf lymph) was

introduced in Britain in the 1880s but even then it was intended that the vaccinators should use it 'for the commencement of a local series of arm to arm vaccinations' (quoted by Hutchinson, 1947, p. 126). However, the advantages of using animal lymph were gradually appreciated and arm-to-arm vaccination was prohibited by the Vaccination Act of 1898. The organization and control of vaccination in other countries was along similar lines although Britain lagged behind in the introduction of animal lymph.

The continued propagation of vaccine by arm-to-arm transfer led to its becoming less effective, and new strains of vaccine were introduced in the mid-nineteenth century. Due to ambiguous statements made by the National Vaccine Establishment it is not possible to determine just how long the original vaccines were kept in use. For example, in their annual report published in April 1838 it was claimed that they were using 'the matter originally collected by Dr Jenner 38 years ago' (National Vaccine Establishment, 1838). It is not clear to which vaccine this referred. Jenner did obtain a vaccine in 1800 from Tanner which was also sent to the Smallpox Hospital, but no great attention was paid to it in the early literature (Baron, 1838, 1, p. 379). If the report published in 1838 is read as referring to the Establishment's activities in 1837, then the vaccine referred to would have been introduced in 1799, and would probably have been either the Bumpus or Kentish Town strain. However, the point is academic because it is extremely unlikely that the original strains were maintained for so long. I have mentioned in Chapter 12 how Jenner sent horsepox strains to the NVE in 1813 and 1817, and in the annual report published in 1839 the directors stated that they 'had taken a good opportunity more than once or twice of recruiting our stores with fresh genuine matter' (National Vaccine Establishment, 1839).

Other vaccines were established privately and distributed very widely. Some, such as those of Badcock and Ceely described earlier, were believed to have been derived from smallpox. Others were believed to have been derived from cowpox. One such strain was introduced in 1838 by John Estlin of Bristol whose findings were published in a series of letters in the *Medical Gazette*. These letters have been gathered together by Crookshank (Crookshank, 1889, II, pp. 323–62). Estlin's vaccine originated from an outbreak in cows. When used in humans it produced a more marked reaction than the vaccines then in use and according to Estlin 'so much resembles the original cow-pox in a more energetic form', and in another letter he described the 'larger and longer-contained areola, more constitutional disturbances, and a much deeper indentation left on the arm' (Crookshank, 1889, II, pp. 328–9). The NVE, who made a small-scale trial of Estlin's vaccine, declined to recommend it but it is clear from Estlin's letters that it was widely used both in Britain and abroad.

According to Gregory, the physician in charge, the Smallpox Hospital had relied on one vaccine strain for many years but had noticed a reduction in its effectiveness. A new strain was introduced in 1838 from an unknown source by Mr Marson which was 'far more intense and active than the strain then in use'. The old strain was discontinued (Gregory, 1838).

Ceely also introduced vaccines derived from infected cows and these were widely used (Ceely, 1842). Crookshank, in the survey of cowpox which led him to believe that it was common, mentioned that a number of vaccines were established in similar circumstances to Ceely's both in Britain and on the Continent, including one by Bousquet which produced severe reactions (Crookshank, 1889, II, pp. 311–22). Because cowpox and related viruses were not enzootic in America, vaccine producers there had to rely on vaccine strains imported from Europe or on vaccines supposedly derived from smallpox. So, during the middle period of the nineteenth century the early vaccine strains were gradually replaced by, or perhaps occasionally mixed with, vaccines isolated from bovine or equine infections and those thought to have been derived from smallpox. Some of these 'second generation' vaccines may have survived into the twentieth century, but the origins of the vaccines used in recent years cannot be identified.

Not all vaccine strains are identical. Some such as the Copenhagen and Tashkent strains produced unacceptably severe reactions and were discontinued. As well as differences in human pathogenicity, differences in laboratory characteristics can also be detected (Fenner, 1958; Baxby, 1975). Many vaccine strains are available for study and have been compared, but the vaccines used since the 1960s were produced from three basic strains. These are the Lister Institute strain from England (sometimes referred to as the Elstree strain), the Wyeth strain from America, and the EM63 strain from Russia. These strains were selected in preference to the others because they produced an adequate level of immunity without producing too severe a local lesion or too high a risk of other complications. The Lister strain was apparently sent to England from Cologne in 1907 (Dudgeon, 1963). It is supposed to have been derived from a case of smallpox in a soldier in the Franco-Prussian war of 1870, although there is no documentary evidence to support this suggestion (personal communication from Professor Colin Kaplan). Before that, the strain from Bordeaux had been used in England and this may well have been one of the equine strains used there (Crookshank, 1889, 1, p. 418). The Wyeth strain was developed from the strain used by the New York Board of Health. According to the records of the New York Health Department, vaccine production was started in 1876 using a strain of vaccine which had been imported from England in 1856 'so we may assume that we started with the Jenner strain' (quoted by Berg and Stevens, 1971). This is a good example of the wishful thinking which probably happened all too often in the nineteenth century. The EM63 strain was developed in Russia from the vaccine used in Ecuador which itself came from the State Health Department in Massachusetts. The origin of the Massachusetts strain is unknown but is believed to have been derived from the New York strain (Anderson, 1969).

The differences between the many vaccine strains are not great, and all strains of vaccinia virus are clearly identifiable as such; none would be mistaken for cowpox or smallpox. Consequently when considering the origins of vaccinia virus we have to decide how such a family of closely related strains may have been derived from the possible parents. The production of a number of similar but not identical vaccines from diverse origins may be explained by the following hypotheses.

1. All have the same 'single parent' origin. This would be cowpox or smallpox or horsepox. The differences seen now among the vaccines would reflect the differences known to exist among the individual strains of the parent, plus any minor differences attributable to different propagation methods. Although horsepox has not been studied by virologists in this century it is probable that not all strains of horsepox virus were identical because strain differences are very common among poxviruses.
2. Different vaccines had different parents, i.e. smallpox, cowpox, horsepox, and genetic hybrids. The differences seen now would reflect the differences between the basic parents in addition to those differences mentioned under the first hypothesis.
3. Different vaccines were originally derived from different parents as in Hypothesis 2. However, during the latter part of the nineteenth century the various attempts which were made to select out the most suitable strains led to the survival only of those derived from one particular parent.

From the circumstances surrounding the introduction of many of the nineteenth-century vaccines I think that the first hypothesis is the least likely. The second hypothesis does not explain why no surviving vaccine has retained any of the properties usually regarded as being characteristic of cowpox or smallpox. The third hypothesis is a compromise between the first two, and explains the survival of a family of closely related vaccines of diverse origins. However, it shares with the second hypothesis the objection that no specifically parental characteristic has survived. This objection may be met by the suggestion that the vaccine strains which have survived through commercial propagation have their origins, not in cowpox or smallpox viruses which have survived naturally, but in the horsepox virus which has been eliminated from its natural habitat. Thus there are four possible origins for modern vaccine strains, namely smallpox, cowpox, horsepox, and hybrids.

The possibility that strains of vaccinia were derived from smallpox has been discussed at length in previous chapters. Although it still remains a possibility I think it is the least likely origin. The production of vaccine by variolation of animals was confidently believed to occur by many, but it has not been achieved in properly controlled modern experiments. The suggestion that vaccines were developed from smallpox by arm-to-arm transfer has always had some strong advocates and the idea has received recent support from Peter Razzell. Perhaps the simplest argument against this theory in general, however, is the fact that successful vaccines with the properties of vaccinia were not developed until Jenner and his contemporaries started to experiment with animal poxviruses. As McVail wrote:

> Indeed I have met with no evidence in the history of inoculation that any such vesicles as pourtrayed [sic] by Jenner, Aikin, and others, had ever before been seen or heard of as a result of any inoculative process (McVail, 1896).

It would be unwise to suggest that no vaccine was ever derived from smallpox, but I believe it likely that smallpox played only a minor role in the development of vaccine strains. Most attention has always been focused on Woodville's vaccinations at the Smallpox Hospital because it was on these strains that the subsequent practice of vaccination was founded. However, as discussed earlier, there is no evidence that smallpox played a significant role in the development of these vaccines. The one patient of Woodville's who has always received particular attention was

Ann Bumpus, probably because she represented a direct link between Woodville and Jenner. However, as described in Chapter 8, a detailed analysis of this case suggests that the vaccine obtained from her was not derived from smallpox. Its most likely constituent was the virus with which the cow was originally infected.

Another possible origin of vaccines is that they were genetic hybrids. Some of the threads distributed by Pearson were almost certainly contaminated with smallpox virus, and mixed infections probably occurred on other occasions. It is in circumstances such as these that hybridization could have occurred. Bedson's and Dumbell's original idea of a hybrid was one whose parents were smallpox and cowpox viruses. However, it is also possible that smallpox and horsepox or horsepox and cowpox could have been the parents. Although some nineteenth-century vaccines may well have been hybrids there is an objection, which will be mentioned later, to the idea that any hybrids have survived into the modern virological era.

The third possible origin for vaccinia is that it was derived from cowpox. Before discussing this possibility something should be said about the relationships of present-day cowpox and vaccinia viruses. If account is taken of their properties and behaviour it is obvious that they are quite distinct. For example, vaccinia strains replicate faster and at higher temperatures than does cowpox. The lesions produced in animals by cowpox are more haemorrhagic than those of vaccinia, and cowpox-infected tissues contain a conspicuous inclusion which is absent from cells infected with vaccinia (Figure 22). There are also antigenic differences which, although insignificant from an immunological point of view, reflect major structural differences (Baxby, 1972). There are also other differences in biological behaviour which are perhaps reflected in differences which have been found in the composition of their structural proteins and DNA (Turner and Baxby, 1979; Esposito et al., 1978; Mackett and Archard, 1979). In fact the differences between vaccinia and cowpox are probably as great as those between vaccinia and smallpox.

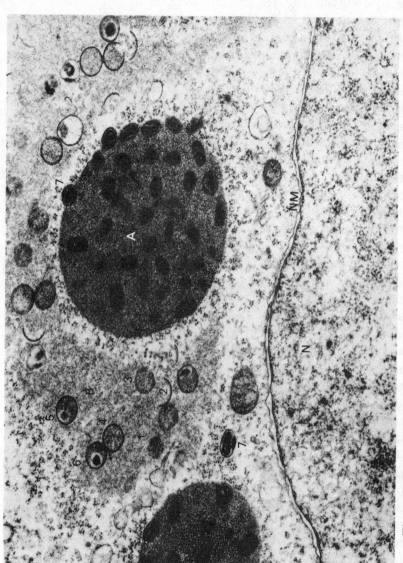

Figure 22 Electronmicrograph of a chick cell infected with cowpox virus. N = nucleus of chick cell, NM = nuclear membrane, A = A-type inclusion produced by cowpox but not smallpox or vaccinia viruses, B = B-type inclusion, produced by all poxviruses, in which virus replication and assembly takes place. Numbers indicate probable sequence of events in virus replication and assembly. (Author's Collection).

Consequently the transformation of cowpox into vaccinia is almost as difficult to envisage as the transformation of smallpox into vaccinia. Cowpox, however, has a wider host range than smallpox and so the initial host range mutant, so important in a vaccine derived from smallpox, would not be necessary.

The assumption has always been made that what the early workers referred to as cowpox was caused by a virus which we would recognize as cowpox virus. The uncertainty about the natural history of cowpox plus the existence of horsepox in the nineteenth century means that this assumption is not necessarily justified. Human infection with cowpox virus is nowadays usually more severe than vaccination but this is not a sufficiently reliable feature to make clinical diagnosis infallible. The only information we have about the possible identity of the viruses being used by the early vaccinators comes from the written descriptions and coloured engravings which have been left. However, there are dangers in trying to make clinical diagnoses from such evidence, and it is possibly unwise to assume that any vaccine which produced a relatively severe reaction contained what we would recognize as cowpox virus. For instance some early vaccines would certainly have been contaminated with pathogenic bacteria and so it is not possible to determine whether a particular vaccine produced a severe reaction because of this contamination or because it contained a more virulent virus. However, it might be reasonable to assume that a vaccine which did not produce a severe reaction was unlikely to be contaminated. One of the greatest problems is the lack of agreement over what constituted a severe reaction. I have discussed (Chapter 6) Jenner's misleading comparisons between cowpox and inoculated smallpox and pointed out that the engravings in his *Inquiry* probably gave the most accurate idea of the lesions produced by his original vaccines. There is also the ambiguity of the different accounts of the effect of the Stonehouse vaccine, and also Crookshank's subjective approach to the subject in his *History*. However, despite all these reservations it is probably worth discussing any apparent differences among the early vaccines, and in particular any difference between the early vaccines on the one hand and later vaccines and cowpox on the other.

There were reports that early vaccines did not all give the same results but as discussed earlier it was the production of generalized eruptions which attracted the most attention. Probably the only direct comparison of the local lesions where a firm conclusion was drawn was the one made by Stromeyer described in Chapter 9. He found that Jenner's vaccine produced a more serious local lesion than Pearson's. Sacco thought that his vaccine produced a less severe local reaction than the English strains. However, his comparison was an indirect one because he had not used English vaccine at that time. Woodville and Pearson did not use Jenner's original strains, and by the time Jenner used their vaccines his original strains were no longer available for direct comparison. Consequently the comparisons were made indirectly and were probably influenced to some extent by hindsight. Woodville drew particular attention to the similarity between his first case of casual cowpox and the case illustrated in Jenner's *Inquiry*, and Jenner thought that the Bumpus strain produced effects similar to the ones depicted in the *Inquiry*. However, Pearson and Woodville soon thought that their London strains produced a more mild effect and were worried by Jenner's use of the term erysipelatous and by his use of caustic to treat the lesions. A little later Pearson admitted that his strains could produce a relatively severe reaction but preferred to refer to it as erythematous. In his analysis of Jenner's Parliamentary Petition, Pearson included an engraved frontispiece showing the vaccine reaction at various intervals after inoculation (Pearson, 1802). The lesion shown in this plate, published at a time when the rift between Pearson and Jenner was at its widest, are very similar to those depicted by Jenner. In fact the same comments apply to other engravings of vaccination published during this period, including those of Paytherus reproduced in Figure 10, and also those published by Aikin (1801), Kirtland (1802), Ballhorn and Stromeyer (1804), and

Willan (1806). These are best appreciated by studying the coloured originals which are not all easily accessible. However, those from Jenner's *Inquiry* and those of Ballhorn and Stromeyer were reproduced in colour by Crookshank whilst McVail reproduced Kirtland's plates, also in colour. The Rev. Holt in the account of his results with one of Pearson's threads noted specifically that 'the appearance and progress were exactly similar to the description and beautiful plate given by Dr Jenner (Holt, 1799). So, although some accounts suggested that there might have been differences among some early vaccines, other accounts, and particularly the illustrated ones, indicated that there was a remarkable similarity in the effects produced by the early vaccines. This does not mean that they had the same origin, but means that there is no clear clinical evidence that they must have had different origins.

Some of the second generation vaccines produced severe reactions and may have contained what we would recognize as cowpox virus. Prime candidates are the vaccines introduced in England by Estlin and Marson, and those isolated in France by Bousquet. On the other hand, although some of the accidental infections investigated and illustrated by Ceely were severe, the viruses isolated from them gave relatively mild reactions when used as vaccines. Ceely made a specific reference to Jenner's illustrations in each of his papers on cowpox. In the first he noted that 'the plate of the casual cowpox on the hand of Sarah Nelmes is a beautiful and faithful delineation of the disease on a fair skin' (Ceely, 1840, p. 334). In his second paper he wrote 'that we have no better standard of comparison of the local and constitutional symptoms of efficient vaccine than that originally furnished and so beautifully illustrated by Jenner' (Ceely, 1842, p. 261). So again we have a similarity between the early mild vaccines and later ones which were supposed to contain cowpox.

The next series of comparisons were made at the end of the nineteenth century. Again the accounts are to some extent contradictory, because we have Creighton at variance with

McVail, and also Crookshank's change of heart (Chapter 10). However, despite the attempts of Creighton and Crookshank to emphasize the loathsomeness of vaccination, it is clear that it was not so very serious. McVail briefly reviewed the illustrations at the time of the Jenner centenary. His main objectives were to discuss the Jenner-Woodville controversy and to publish the plates made by Kirtland which were thought not to have been published before. McVail was struck by the similarity among the different early vaccines, and also by the similarities between the early vaccines on the one hand and the late nineteenth-century strains on the other. Of the effects of the early vaccines he wrote, 'The appearance shown in the plates in question were those of vaccinia as we still know it . . . The same appearance can still be seen at the present time by any medical man who watches the course of one of his own cases. The vaccination of 1802 is identical with the vaccination of 1896, and there is cultivation neither upward nor downwards' (McVail, 1896).

The similarities between the earliest vaccines and those of the late nineteenth century can be extended to those of today by comparing Figures 6, 7, and 10 with Figure 11. I have identified, above, the sources of coloured illustrations of early vaccination lesions, and coloured illustrations of modern vaccination lesions have been published by Emond (1974), from which Figure 11 is taken, and also by Smadel (1952), and Dixon (1962).

The foregoing brief survey emphasizes the remarkable similarity between most of the early vaccines and those of the mid- and late-nineteenth century and those of today, and also shows that they were characterized by a relative mildness. Consequently there is no need to assume on clinical grounds that the earliest vaccines must have necessarily contained viruses different to the ones used today. However, it is likely that some vaccines contained cowpox and it is possible that the strains introduced by such as Estlin, Marson, and Bousquet might have come into this category. If this was so then they must have either been discontinued or become transformed into vaccinia.

Opinions have differed on the possibility that vaccines were developed from cowpox. Crookshank and Creighton thought that it was impossible because they believed that there was no immunological relationship between smallpox and cowpox. Razzell, although maintaining that the Woodville-Pearson vaccines were derived from smallpox, suggested that Jenner's early strains and some later strains such as those of Estlin and Ceely's bovine strains were cowpox. The differences between present-day cowpox and vaccinia have been summarized. Allan Downie, the first to distinguish between the two viruses, emphasizes their similarities and believes that cowpox is the most likely source of vaccinia (Downie, 1970). On the other hand Fritz Dekking of Amsterdam, who has isolated and studied many strains of cowpox and bovine vaccinia in Holland, emphasizes their differences and believes it 'improbable' that vaccinia was derived from cowpox. Unfortunately he did not give his own view of the likely origin and was content to leave the problem unsolved (Dekking, 1964). I believe that any vaccines derived from cowpox would have tended to produce too severe reactions and would have been replaced by more suitable strains. The alternative, that they did undergo the necessarily long and gradual transformation into vaccinia, I too find improbable.

There is one striking feature about present-day comparisons of smallpox, cowpox, and vaccinia viruses which led me to consider another possible origin for vaccinia. It is that none of the many strains of vaccinia which have survived have any of the properties thought of as being characteristic of cowpox or smallpox. If any of these vaccines had been derived from cowpox or smallpox some of them should have retained some characteristic more usually associated with the parent. If any vaccines were hybrids they might be expected to have some characteristics of both parents. However, this has not happened. The vaccines which proved most successful and which have continued in use into the twentieth century behaved in a manner remarkably similar to that of the early vaccines, and make up a very closely related group of viruses quite distinct from smallpox and cowpox viruses. It is therefore reasonable to suggest that they had an origin independent of these viruses. If this is so, it is tempting to suggest that they may represent the horsepox which was eliminated from its natural habitat at the end of the nineteenth century. We know that strains of vaccine were established from infected horses on various occasions throughout the nineteenth century both in England and on the Continent, and Jenner believed that his cowpox originated in horses. It must also be remembered that there is no certainty that cowpox as we know it ever was enzootic in cows. Horsepox could infect cows and it is possible that some of the vaccines established from cows in fact contained horsepox. Although Loy, Lafont, and Sacco suggested that horsepox tended to produce a relatively severe reaction when passed directly from horse to man, the typical vaccine reaction very soon established itself. So there is no clinical reason why some of the early vaccines should not have contained a horsepox virus which we would have recognized as vaccinia.

Unfortunately virtually nothing is known about the inter-relationships between cowpox and vaccinia on the one hand and horsepox on the other, except for one tantalizing piece of evidence supplied by Sacco. In 1966 Anton Mayr, one of Herrlich's colleagues in Munich, showed that hens could be infected with vaccinia whereas cowpox had no effect. Mayr proposed that this test should be used as a simple means of distinguishing between the two viruses and the method has been used consistently by those trained by the Munich workers. In 1809 Sacco published a treatise on vaccination in which he summarized various attempts to vaccinate animals. In it he recorded that some workers, unfortunately not identified, succeeded in infecting hens with vaccine (Sacco, 1809, p. 178). If this result is taken at face value it indicates a closer relationship between some early vaccines and the ones used today than between those early vaccines and present-day cowpox strains.

I had hoped that the earliest studies on the histology of

viral inclusions in infected cells would provide some information. However, these observations were concerned with investigating the protozoal nature of viruses, and the illustrations made by these early workers reflect their attempts to prove or disprove this particular theory. The characteristic inclusion which would be expected to be absent in smallpox-infected tissues and present in tissues infected with cowpox is not recognizable in these early studies. Neither, unfortunately, is it recognizable in studies on fowlpox virus, which also produces typical inclusions (Bollinger, 1873; Guarnieri, 1892; Sanfelice, 1897). Consequently no valid conclusions can be drawn from these studies.

The idea that some vaccines were derived from horsepox was widely accepted in the nineteenth century, but that vaccinia may be equated with horsepox is an idea that has not been considered by modern medical historians and virologists. Certainly the suggestion is supported by very little evidence. However, it seems to be the inevitable conclusion if we accept as improbable the idea that cowpox or smallpox could be transformed into a third, quite distinct virus. Although virus mutants are well known, usually very few characters are changed, and the mutants are clearly recognizable as variants of the parents. There is no precedent in virology for the transformation of one virus into another. In 1978 Russian workers reported that they had isolated mutants of monkeypox virus which were indistinguishable from smallpox virus (Marennikova and Shelukhina, 1978). However, mutants of monkeypox had been recognized earlier and those isolated by the Russian workers are not yet sufficiently characterized to suggest that they are more than superficially similar to smallpox.

The analyses of poxvirus DNA published by Mackett and Archard (1979) have recently been subjected to a so far unpublished computer analysis by Frank Fenner. This shows that smallpox, cowpox, and vaccinia are quite distinct and Fenner suggests that it is most unlikely that any one virus could have been derived from the others. It has also been suggested that all poxviruses may have developed from one primitive ancestor. In this case the time taken for the different viruses to emerge with their own specific characteristics would be measured on an evolutionary time scale, and would take much longer than the very short periods in which cowpox or smallpox would have had in which to transform into vaccinia. Indeed the use of the term transformation implies an unusually rapid and unexpected event.

It has been said that the origins of vaccinia will never be known. This is true, and for many people this is part of the fascination because it means that no reasonable hypothesis can be disproved. All that one can do is analyse the early literature in the light of present-day information. It is unlikely that future studies on the viruses will provide any further important information on the subject because work on smallpox virus is now severely restricted. Although smallpox has been eradicated, antigenically related poxviruses still circulate in their appropriate reservoirs, and any threat to future human populations will come from these animal poxviruses. For instance the eradication of smallpox from West Africa has revealed that monkeypox can cause a disease in man which resembles smallpox, but fortunately with little or no potential for case-to-case spread (Arita, 1979). Only time will tell whether the process of evolution will lead to the re-emergence of smallpox virus, perhaps from monkeypox or some other related virus. If this does happen the time taken will again be measured on the evolutionary time scale. It is the possibility that this might happen in the distant future which makes it important for fundamental studies on smallpox virus to continue, but only the most essential work with smallpox virus will be done in a handful of reference laboratories. Research into animal poxviruses will continue but the experiments required to prove or disprove the origin of vaccinia from smallpox will almost certainly never be done.

In summary I think that not all the nineteenth-century vaccines had the same origin. The least likely possibility is that they were derived from smallpox, and certainly the famous Bumpus strain was unlikely to have been derived in this way. Some vaccines were probably derived from what we would now recognize as cowpox, some from horsepox, and some were probably hybrids. However, the vaccines studied in the twentieth century have none of the specific characteristics usually associated with cowpox or smallpox and form a homogeneous group in their own right. Apart from occasionally severe exceptions the appearance of the vaccination lesion has remained remarkably constant since 1796. My objective in starting this book was to review the evidence in the light of up-to-date information without necessarily coming to a particular conclusion. However, my own opinion is that the occasionally severe vaccines which were introduced in the nineteenth century were probably derived from cowpox or hybrids and were discontinued, whereas the closely related family of surviving strains probably represent the missing horsepox. Jenner would certainly recognize today's vaccines as being indistinguishable from the ones he used, and I would like to think that the early vaccines contained what we would now recognize as vaccinia virus.

What of the leading characters in all this?

The practice of vaccination was certainly put on a firm basis by the work of people such as Woodville and Pearson in England, and Sacco and de Carro on the Continent. Had Woodville and Pearson not found a source of vaccine in London so soon after the publication of Jenner's *Inquiry*, and carried out their own very extensive trials, it is possible that there would have been considerable delay before vaccination became established. In fact, so critical of Jenner were some of the early comments that it needed someone with the drive of Pearson and the facilities available to Woodville at the Smallpox Hospital in order to generate the necessary impetus. Nevertheless the important fact is that they were only applying the principle which Jenner had put forward.

Writers have always found it difficult to be objective about Jenner. Too often he has been depicted as the genius seen by Baron or the charlatan depicted by Creighton. Obviously the truth lies between these two extremes. Perhaps Jenner had only two faults, and for neither can he be held responsible; he was human, and his ideas on vaccination were far in advance of contemporary medical thought. Although the actual work on which his theories were based was limited this should not detract from their soundness or his vision. Perhaps the closest he came to genius can best be seen in his recognition and explanation of true and spurious cowpox. However, the basic and most important theory was that an animal poxvirus, whatever its actual identity, would protect against smallpox, and this theory has been amply confirmed. How far Jenner was ahead of his time can be appreciated from three simple facts.

1. It was not until the 1880s that Louis Pasteur introduced the next immunizing agents.
2. It was 1921 before the first live bacterial vaccine for general human use was introduced – BCG vaccine for tuberculosis.
3. It was not until the late 1950s that the second live virus vaccine for general human use was introduced – the Sabin vaccine for poliomyelitis.

The possibility that smallpox could be eradicated had been suggested before the introduction of vaccination, for example by John Haygarth. With the development of effective smallpox vaccine that hope became a reality and smallpox has been eradicated. It is perhaps ironic that the origins of the vaccine which played such an important role in this achievement may always remain a mystery, despite all the attention which has been paid to the topic since 1798.

Literature Cited

Abraham, J. J., *Lettsom, his Life, Times, Friends and Descendants* (London: Heinemann, 1933), p. 351.

Adams, J., *Observations on Morbid Poisons* (London: Johnson, 1795).

Adams, J., *A Popular View of the Vaccine Inoculation* (London: Phillips, 1807).

Aikin, C. R., *A Concise View of all the most Important Facts which have hitherto appeared concerning the Cow-pox* (London: Phillips, 1801).

Anderson, E. K., Selection of a strain of vaccinia virus for production of smallpox vaccine, in *Symposium on Smallpox* (Zagreb: Yugoslav Academy of Sciences and Arts, 1969), pp. 53–64.

Arita, I., Virological evidence for the success of the smallpox eradication programme, *Nature*, 1979, **279,** 293–8.

Arita, I. and Henderson, D. A., Smallpox and monkeypox in non-human primates, *Bull. WHO*, 1968, **39,** 277–83.

Baker, G., *An Inquiry into the Merits of a Method of Inoculating the Smallpox* (London: Dodsley, 1766).

Ballhorn, G. F. and Stromeyer, C., *Traité de l'Inoculation* (Leipzig: Reclam, 1804).

Baron, J., *Life of Edward Jenner* (London: Colborn, 1838, 2 vols).

Barry, F. W., *Report of an Epidemic of Smallpox at Sheffield, 1887–8* (London: HMSO, 1889).

Bauer, D. J., St Vincent, L., Kempe, C. H., Young, P. A. and Downie, A. W., Prophylaxis of smallpox with Methisazone, *Am. J. Epid.*, 1969, **90**, 130–45.

Baxby, D., A comparison of the antigens present on the surface of virus released artificially from chick cells infected with vaccinia virus and cowpox virus and its white pock mutant, *J. Hyg.*, 1972, **70**, 353–65.

Baxby, D., Identification and interrelationships of the variola-vaccinia subgroup of poxviruses, *Prog. Med. Virol.*, 1975, **19**, 215–46.

Baxby, D., Is cowpox misnamed? A review of ten human cases, *Brit. Med. J.*, 1977a, **i**, 1379–81.

Baxby, D., Poxvirus hosts and reservoirs, *Archives Virol.*, 1977b, **55**, 169–79.

Baxby, D., An unusual portrait of Edward Jenner and a possible link with Napoleon, *Med. Hist.*, 1978, **22**, 335–9.

Baxby, D., Edward Jenner, William Woodville, and the origins of vaccinia virus, *J. Hist. Med.*, 1979, **34**, 134–62.

Baxby, D., Ashton, D. G., Jones, D., Thomsett, L. R. and Denham, E. M., Cowpox virus from unusual hosts, *Vet. Rec.*, 1979, **109**, 175.

Baxby, D. and Osborne, A. D., Antibody studies in natural bovine cowpox, *J. Hyg.*, 1979, **83**, 425–9.

Bedson, H. S. and Dumbell, K. R., Hybrids derived from the viruses of variola major and cowpox, *J. Hyg.*, 1964, **62**, 147–58.

Bedson, H. S. and Dumbell, K. R., Smallpox and vaccinia, *Brit. Med. Bull.*, 1967, **23**, 119–23.

Berg, T. O. and Stevens, D. A., *Catalogue of Viruses, Rickettsiae, Chlamydiae* (Rockville: American Type Culture Collection, 4th edition, 1971).

Bevan, E., Correspondence, *Med. Phys. J.*, 1801, **5**, 455–6.

Bishop, W. J., Thomas Dimsdale, MD, FRS (1712–1800) and the inoculation of Catharine the Great of Russia, *Ann. Med. Hist.*, n.s., 1932, **4**, 321–38.

Blaxall, F. R., Report on equine variola, in *Annual Report of the Local Government Board, 1901–2* (London: HMSO, 1903), pp. 568–9.

Blaxall, F. R., Smallpox; Animal pock diseases, in *A System of Bacteriology in Relation to Medicine* (London: HMSO, 1930), vol. 7, pp. 84–132, 140–56.

Bollinger, O. von, Uber Epithelioma contagiosum beim Haushuhn und die sogenannten Pocken des Geflügels, *Virchow's Arch. Path. Anat. Phys.*, 1873, **58**, 349–61.

British Medical Journal, Jenner Centenary Number, 1896, **i**, 1246–312.

Bulloch, W., Obituary – Charles Creighton, *Lancet*, 1927, **ii**, 250–1.

Carro, J. de, Correspondence, *Med. Phys. J.*, 1803, **9**, 450–7.

Ceely, R., Observations on the variolae vaccinae, *Trans. Prov. Med. Surg. Assoc.*, 1840, **8**, 287–435.

Ceely, R., Further observations on the variolae vaccinae, *Trans. Prov. Med. Surg. Assoc.*, 1842, **10**, 209–76.

Chandler, B., *An Essay towards an Investigation of the Present Successful and Most General Method of Inoculation* (London: Wilkie, 1767).

Chauveau, A., Sur la transformation des virus à propos des relations qui existent entre la vaccine et la variole, *Bull. Acad. Méd.*, 1891, **26**, 498–519, 565–80.

Christie, A. B., *Infectious Diseases* (Edinburgh and London: Livingstone, 1969).

Christie, T., Correspondence, *Med. Phys. J.*, 1805, **13**, 122–8.

Condamine, C. M. de la, *A Discourse on Inoculation* (London: Vaillant, 1755).

Cooke, C., Correspondence, in *Contributions to Physical and Medical Knowledge*, ed. T. Beddoes (Bristol: Longman, 1799), pp. 387–98.

Copeman, S. A. M., *Vaccination, its Natural History and Pathology* (London: MacMillan, 1899).

Copeman, S. A. M., The inter-relationship of variola and vaccinia, *Proc. Roy. Soc.*, 1903, **71**, 121–33.

Copeman, S. A. M., Report of the investigation of an

outbreak of cow-pox on a farm at Buckland near Reigate, in *Annual Report of the Local Government Board, 1902–3* (London: HMSO, 1904), Supplement, pp. 258–66.

Creighton, C., *The Natural History of Cowpox and Vaccinial Syphilis* (London: Cassell, 1887).

Creighton, C., *Jenner and Vaccination* (London: Sonnenschein, 1889).

Creighton, C., *A History of Epidemics in Britain* (London: Cass, 2nd edition, 1965, 2 vols).

Crookshank, E. M., *Manual of Bacteriology* (London: Lewis, 2nd edition, 1887).

Crookshank, E. M., An investigation of an outbreak of cow-pox in Wiltshire, *Brit. Med. J.*, 1888, **i**, 1–5, 63–8.

Crookshank, E. M., *History and Pathology of Vaccination* (London: Lewis, 1889, 2 vols).

Crummer, L. R., Copy of Jenner notebook, *Ann. Med. Hist.*, n.s., 1929, **1**, 403–48.

Dekking, F., Cowpox and vaccinia, in *Zoonoses*, ed. J. van der Hoeden (London: Elsevier, 1964).

Dick, G., Routine smallpox vaccination, *Brit. Med. J.*, 1971, **ii**, 163–6.

Dimsdale, T., *The Present Method of Inoculating for the Smallpox* (London: Owen, 5th edition, 1769).

Dimsdale, T., *Remarks on a Letter to Sir Robert Barker, and George Stackpole upon General Inoculation by John Coakley Lettsom* (London: Phillips, 1779).

Dimsdale, T., *Tracts on Inoculation written and published at St Petersburgh in the year 1768* (London: Phillips, 1781).

Dixon, C. W., *Smallpox* (London: Churchill, 1962).

Downie, A. W., A study of the lesions produced experimentally by cowpox virus, *J. Path. Bact.*, 1939, **48**, 361–79.

Downie, A. W., The immunological relationship of the virus of spontaneous cowpox to vaccinia virus, *Brit. J. Exp. Path.*, 1939, **20**, 158–76.

Downie, A. W., The poxvirus group, in *Viral and Rickettsial*

Infections of Man, ed. by F. L. Horsfall and I. Tamm (Philadelphia: Lippincott, 4th edition, 1965).

Downie, A. W., Smallpox, in *Infectious Agents and Host Reactions*, ed. by S. Mudd (Philadelphia: Saunders, 1970), pp. 487–518.

Drewitt, F. D., *The Notebook of Edward Jenner in the Possession of the Royal College of Physicians of London* (London: OUP, 1931).

Drewitt, F. D., *The Life of Edward Jenner* (London: Longmans, 1931).

Dudgeon, J. A., Development of smallpox vaccine in England in the eighteenth and nineteenth centuries, *Brit. Med. J.*, 1963, **i**, 1367–72.

Dumbell, K. R. and Bedson, H. S., Adaptation of variola virus to growth in the rabbit, *J. Path. Bact.*, 1966, **91**, 459–65.

Dumbell, K. R., Bedson, H. S. and Nizamuddin, M., Thermo-efficient strains of variola major virus, *J. gen. Virol.*, 1967, **1**, 379–81.

Dunning, R., Correspondence, *Med. Phys. J.*, 1803, **10**, 339–45.

Emond, R. T. D., *A Colour Atlas of Infectious Diseases* (London: Wolfe Medical Publications, 1974).

Esposito, J. J., Obijeski, J. F. and Nakano, J. H., Orthopoxvirus DNA: strain differentiation by electrophoresis of restriction endonuclease fragmented virion DNA, *Virology*, 1978, **89**, 53–66.

Evans, J., Correspondence, *Med. Phys. J.*, 1799, **2**, 310–13.

Fenner, F., The biological characteristics of several strains of vaccinia, cowpox and rabbitpox viruses, *Virology*, 1958, **5**, 502–29.

Fenner, F., *Smallpox and its Eradication* (Geneva: WHO, in press).

Finch, W., Correspondence, *Med. Phys. J.*, 1800, **3**, 415–20.

Fisk, D., *Dr. Jenner of Berkeley* (London: Heinemann, 1959).

Foege, W. H., Millar, J. D. and Henderson, D. A., Smallpox

eradication in West and Central Africa, *Bull. WHO*, 1975, **52**, 209–22.

Fraser, H., Observations on the vaccine inoculation, *Med. Chirurg. Trans.*, 1805–6, **12**, 282–6.

Gibbs, E. P. J., Johnson, R. H. and Collings, D. H., Cowpox in a dairy herd in the United Kingdom, *Vet. Rec.*, 1973, **92**, 56–64.

Gibbs, E. P. J., Johnson, R. H. and Osborne, A. D., The differential diagnosis of viral skin infections of the bovine teat, *Vet. Rec.*, 1970, **87**, 602–9.

Gibbs, E. P. J. and Osborne, A. D., Observations on the epidemiology of pseudocowpox in South-West England and South Wales, *Brit. Vet. J.*, 1974, **130**, 150–9.

Gins, H. A., Unitarische oder dualistische Auffassung der Variola-Vaccine?, *Reichs-Gesundh Bl.*, 1938, **11**, 201.

Gispen, R. and Brand-Saathof, B., Three specific antigens produced in vaccinia, variola and monkeypox infections, *J. Inf. Dis.*, 1974, **129**, 289–95.

Greenwood, M., *Epidemic and Crowd Diseases* (London: Williams & Norgate, 1935), pp. 245–73.

Gregory, G., Correspondence, *Lond. Med. Phys. J.*, 1822, **48**, 190–5.

Gregory, G., Report of the smallpox and vaccination hospital, *London Med. Gaz.*, 1838, **21**, 860–2.

Guarnieri, G., Ricerche sulla patogenesi ed etiologia dell' infezione vaccinica e vaiolosa, *Arch. Sci. Med.*, 1892, **16**, 403–23.

Guillou, F.-A., Expériences sur l'inoculation de la vario-loide, *J. Gén. Méd.*, 1827, **98**, 239–41.

Guy, W. A., Two hundred and fifty years of smallpox in London, *J. Roy. Statist. Soc.*, 1882, **45**, 399–433.

Harper, L., Bedson, H. S. and Buchan, A., Identification of orthopoxviruses by polyacrylamide gel electrophoresis of intracellular polypeptides, *Virology*, 1979, **93**, 435–44.

Haygarth, J., *An Inquiry how to prevent the Smallpox* (London: Johnson, 1785).

Haygarth, J., *Sketch of a Plan to exterminate the Casual*

Smallpox from Great Britain and to Introduce General Inoculation (London: Johnson, 1793, 2 vols).

Hellman, C. D., An unpublished diary of Edward Jenner, *Ann. Med. Hist.*, n.s., 1931, **3**, 412–38.

Henderson, D. A., The eradication of smallpox, *Sci. Am.*, 1976a, **235**, 25–33.

Henderson, D. A., Surveillance of smallpox, *Int. J. Epid.*, 1976b, **5**, 19–28.

Herrlich, A., Mayr, A., Mahnel, H. and Munz, E., Experimental studies on transformation of the variola virus into the vaccinia virus, *Archiv. ges. Virusf.*, 1963, **12**, 579–99.

Hime, T. W., Successful transformation of smallpox into cowpox, *Brit. Med. J.*, 1892, **ii**, 117–20.

Hime, T. W., Animal inoculation, *Brit. Med. J.*, 1896, **i**, 1279–89.

Holt, R., Correspondence, *Med. Phys. J.*, 1799, **2**, 401–4.

Horgan, E. S., The experimental transformation of variola to vaccinia, *J. Hyg.*, 1938, **38**, 702–15.

Hughes, T., Correspondence, *Med. Phys. J.*, 1799, **1**, 318–23.

Hungerford, T. G., *Diseases of Livestock* (Auckland: McGraw-Hill, 8th edition, 1975), p. 760.

Hutchinson, J. R., A historical note on the prevention of smallpox in England, in *Report of the Ministry of Health for the Year Ending 31 March 1946* (London: HMSO, 1947), pp. 119–30.

Jenner, E., Observations on the natural history of the cuckoo, unpublished manuscript, 1787, *Royal Society Guard Book 82, Decade IX, Paper 37*.

Jenner, E., Observations on the natural history of the cuckoo, *Phil. Trans. Roy. Soc.*, 1788, **78**, 219–37.

Jenner, E., A process for preparing pure emetic tartar by recrystallization, *Trans. Soc. Imp. Med. Chirurg. Knowl.*, 1793, **1**, 30–3.

Jenner, E., *An Inquiry into the Causes and Effects of the Variolae Vaccinae* (London: Sampson Low, 1798).

Jenner, E., *Further Observations on the Variolae Vaccinae* (London: Sampson Low, 1799).

Jenner, E., Correspondence, *Med. Phys. J.*, 1800a, **3**, 101–2.

Jenner, E., *A Continuation of Facts and Observations relative to the Variolae Vaccinae or Cow Pox* (London: Sampson Low, 1800b).

Jenner, E., *The Origin of the Vaccine Inoculation* (London: Shury, 1801).

Jenner, E., Correspondence, *Med. Phys. J.*, 1804, **12**, 97–102.

Jenner, E., Vaccination. Dr Jenner's circular to the medical profession, *Ed. Med. Surg. J.*, 1821, **17**, 476–8.

Jenner, E., An inquiry into the natural history of a disease known as the cow-pox, *Lancet*, 1923, **i**, 137–41.

Jenner, G., *The Evidence at Large, as laid before the Committee of the House of Commons, respecting Dr Jenner's Discovery of the Vaccine Inoculation* (London: Murray, 1805).

Kelsch, L. F. A., Teissier, P., Camus, L., Tanon, L. et Duvoir, M., De la variole-vaccine. Recherches expéri-mentales présentées à l'Académie de Médécine, *Bull. Acad. Méd.*, 1909, **62**, 13–22.

Kelsch, L. F. A., Teissier, P., Camus, L., Tanon, L. et Duvoir, M., Novelles recherches expérimentales sur la variole-vaccine, *Bull. Acad. Méd.*, 1910, **64**, 92–8.

Kelson, T. M., Correspondence, *Med. Phys. J.*, 1800, **4**, 21–4.

Kirtland, G., *Thirty Plates of Small Pox and Cow Pox drawn from Nature* (London: Johnson, 1802).

Klein, E., On the etiology of vaccinia and variola, in *Annual Report of the Local Government Board for 1892–3* (London: HMSO, 1894), Supplement, pp. 391–412.

Lauder, I. M., Martin, W. B., Murray, M. and Pirie, H. M., Experimental vaccinia infection of cattle: a comparison with other virus infections of cows' teats, *Vet. Rec.*, 1971, **89**, 571–8.

Lawrence, J., On the origin of the cowpox with a few remarks on the pox of swine, *Med. Phys. J.*, 1799, **1**, 114–18.

Le Fanu, W., *A Bio-bibliography of Edward Jenner* (London: Harvey & Blyth, 1951).

Letters. *Letters from the Past, from John Hunter to Edward Jenner* (London: Royal College of Surgeons, 1976).

Lettsom, J. C., Correspondence, *Med. Phys. J.*, 1800, **3**, 567.

Loy, J., *An Account of Some Experiments on the Origin of the Cow Pox* (London: Phillips, 1801).

Mackett, M. and Archard, L. C., Conservation and variation in orthopoxvirus genome structure, *J. gen. Virol.*, 1979, **45**, 683–701.

Marennikova, S. S. and Shelukhina, E. M., Whitepox virus isolated from hamsters inoculated with monkeypox virus, *Nature*, 1978, **276**, 291–2.

Martin, W. B., Martin, B., Hay, D. and Lauder, I. M., Bovine ulcerative mammillitis caused by a herpesvirus, *Vet. Rec.*, 1966, **78**, 494–7.

Martindale, *Martindale's Extra Pharmacopoeia* (London: Pharmaceutical Press, 27th edition, 1971), pp. 1371–2.

Mayr, A., Eine einfache und schnelle Methode zur Differenzierung zwischen Vaccine – (poxvirus officinale) und Kuhpockenvirus – (poxvirus bovis) *Zbl. Bakt. I. Orig.*, 1966, **199**, 144–51.

McConnell, S. J., Herman, Y. F., Mattson, D. E. and Erickson, L., Monkeypox disease in irradiated cynomologus monkeys, *Nature*, 1962, **195**, 1128–9.

McVail, J. C., Cowpox and smallpox: Jenner, Woodville and Pearson, *Brit. Med. J.*, 1896, **i**, 1271–6.

Miller, G., *The Adoption of Inoculation of Smallpox in England and France* (Philadelphia: University of Pennsylvania Press, 1957).

Miller, G., Eighteenth-century attempts to attenuate smallpox virus, *Actes du VIIIe Congrès d'Histoire des Sciences* (Florence, 1958), pp. 804–10.

Monro, A., *Observations on the Different Kinds of Smallpox* (Edinburgh: Constable, 1818).

Monro, A., Observations on the causes of the prevalence of smallpox and on the means of preventing the dissemination of that disease, *Edin. J. Med. Sci.*, 1826, **1**, 280–5.

Moore, J., *The History of the Smallpox* (London: Longmans, 1815).

National Vaccine Establishment, *Report of the Case of the Hon. Robert Grosvenor* (London, 1811).

National Vaccine Establishment, *Copy of the last Report from the National Vaccine Establishment* (London: HMSO, 1838).

National Vaccine Establishment, *Copy of the last Report from the National Vaccine Establishment* (London: HMSO, 1839).

Noehden, A. A., Correspondence, *Med. Phys. J.*, 1803, **9**, 434–8.

O'Malley, J., The original vaccine inoculator, *M. and B. Bull.*, 1954, 129–39.

Parry, C. H., *An Inquiry into the Symptoms and Causes of the Syncope Anginosa* (London: Cadell & Davies, 1799).

Paul, H., *The Control of Diseases* (Edinburgh and London: Livingstone, 1964).

Paytherus, T., *A Comparative Statement of Facts and Observations Relative to the Cow Pox* (London: Shury, 2nd edition, 1801).

Pearson, G., *An Inquiry Concerning the History of the Cow Pox* (London: Johnson, 1798).

Pearson, G., Circular letter, *Med. Phys. J.*, 1799a, **1**, 113–14.

Pearson, G., A statement of the progress in the vaccine inoculation, *Med. Phys. J.*, 1799b, **2**, 213–25.

Pearson, G., A communication concerning eruptions resembling the smallpox which sometimes appear in the vaccine disease, *Med. Phys. J.*, 1800a, **3**, 97–101.

Pearson, G., Correspondence, *Med. Phys. J.*, 1800b, **3**, 411–12.

Pearson, G., *An Examination of the Report of the Committee of the House of Commons on the Claims of Remuneration for the Vaccine Pock Inoculation* (London: Johnson, 1802).

Razzell, P. E., Edward Jenner: the history of a medical myth, *Med. Hist.*, 1965 **9**, 216–29.

Razzell, P. E., *Edward Jenner's Cowpox Vaccine: the History of a Medical Myth* (Firle: Caliban, 1977a).

Razzell, P. E., *The Conquest of Smallpox* (Firle: Caliban, 1977b).

Redfearn, R., Correspondence, *Med. Phys. J.*, 1799, **2**, 23–5.

Report, *The Present State of Vaccination* (London: HMSO, 1840).

Rhazes, A Treatise on the Smallpox and Measles (London: New Sydenham Society, 1848).

Ricketts, T. F. and Byles, J. B., *The Diagnosis of Smallpox* (London: Cassell, 1908).

Ring, J., Correspondence, *Med. Phys. J.*, 1799, **2**, 25–9.

Ring, J., Correspondence, *Lond. Med. Rev.*, 1800, **3**, 314.

Ring, J., *A Treatise on the Cowpox* (London: Carpenter & Johnson, 1801).

Ring, J., Correspondence, *Med. Phys. J.*, 1802, **7**, 109–11.

Ringer, S. and Sainsbury, H., *Handbook of Therapeutics* (London: Lewis, 13th edition, 1897), pp. 187–9.

Rosenwald, C. D., Variolation and other observations made during a smallpox epidemic in the southern province of Tanganyika, *Med. Off.*, 1951, **85**, 87–90.

Royal Commission, *Vaccination and its Results, a Report based on the Evidence taken by the Royal Commission* (London: New Sydenham Society, 1898).

Ruston, T., *An Essay on Inoculation for the Smallpox* (London: Dilly & Payne, 1768).

Sacco, L., *Osservazioni Pratiche sull'uso de Vajuolo Vaccino, come Preservativo de Vajuolo Umano* (Milan: Sacco, 1801).

Sacco, L., Review, *Med. Phys. J.*, 1802, **7**, 169–85.

Sacco, L., *Trattato di Vaccinazione con Osservazioni sul Giavardo e Vajuolo Pecorino* (Milan: Mussi, 1809).

Sanfelice, F., U@ber die pathogene Wirkung der Blastomyceten, *Z. Hyg. Infekt. Krankh.*, 1897, **26**, 257–81.

Saunders, P. L., Edward Jenner: the Cheltenham years, *Practitioner*, 1969, **203**, 225–30.

Simon, J., *Papers Relating to the History and Practice of Vaccination* (London: HMSO, 1857).

Sims, J., Correspondence, *Med. Phys. J.*, 1799, **1**, 11–12.

Smadel, J. E., Smallpox and vaccinia, in *Viral and Rickettsial Infections of Man*, ed. T. M. Rivers (Philadelphia: Lippincott, 2nd edition, 1952), pp. 414–39.

Smith, M. H., The 'Real Expedición Maritima de la Vacuna' in New Spain and Guatemala, *Trans. Am. Phil. Soc.*, n.s., 1974, **64**, pt 1.

Stearn, E. W. and Stearn, A. E., *The Effect of Smallpox on the Destiny of the Amerindian* (Boston: Humphries, 1945).

Stevenson, J., Correspondence, *Med. Phys. J.*, 1801, **6**, 121–4.

Stevenson, J., Correspondence, *Med. Phys. J.*, 1802, **7**, 9–11.

Stromeyer, C., Correspondence, *Med. Phys. J.*, 1800, **3**, 471–3.

Sutton, D., *The Inoculator, or Suttonian System of Inoculation* (London: Gillet, 1796).

Teissier, P., Duvoir, M. et Stevenin, Expériences de variolisation sur les singes, *Compt. rends. hebd. Soc. Biol.*, 1911, **70**, 654–6.

Teissier, P., Rivalier, E., Reilly, J. et Stefanesco, V., Essais de transformation variolo-vaccinale à l'aide du virus variolique pur, *Compt. rends. hebd. Soc. Biol.*, 1931, **108**, 1105–7.

Thomson, J., Some observations on the varioloid disease, *Ed. Med. J.*, 1818, **14**, 518–27.

Thornton, E., Correspondence, in *Contributions to Physical and Medical Knowledge*, ed. T. Beddoes (Bristol: Longman, 1799), pp. 398–402.

Trousseau, A., *Lectures on Clinical Medicine* (London: New Sydenham Society, 1869).

→Turner, A. and Baxby, D., Structural polypeptides of *Orthopoxvirus*: their distribution in various members and location within the virion, *J. gen. Virol.*, 1979, **45**, 537–45.

Underwood, E. A., Edward Jenner, Benjamin Waterhouse,

and the introduction of vaccination into the United States, *Nature*, 1949, **163**, 823–8.

Viborg, E., Experiments made for the purpose of proving that the smallpox is a disease common both to man and brutes, *Med. Phys. J.*, 1802, **8**, 271–3.

Ward, M., Correspondence, *Med. Phys. J.*, 1799, **2**, 134–9.

Waterhouse, B., Correspondence, *Med. Phys. J.*, 1801, **6**, 327–31.

Wehrle, P. F., Posch, J., Richter, K. H. and Henderson, D. A., An airborne outbreak of smallpox in a German hospital and its significance with respect to other recent outbreaks, *Bull. WHO*, 1970, **43**, 669–79.

WHO, *WHO Expert Committee on Smallpox Eradication, Second Report* (Geneva: WHO, 1972).

Whyte, D., Correspondence, *Med. Phys. J.*, 1801, **5**, 243–5.

Willan, R., *On Vaccine Inoculation* (London: Phillips, 1806).

Willan, R., *On Cutaneous Diseases* (London: Johnson, 1808).

Williams, G., *Virus Hunters* (London: Hutchinson, 1963), pp. 14–15.

Winslow, O. E., *A Destroying Angel: the Conquest of Smallpox in Colonial Boston* (Boston: Houghton Mifflin, 1974).

Winterburn, G. W., *The Value of Vaccination* (Philadelphia: Boericke, 1886).

Woodville, W., *Medical Botany* (London: Phillips, 4 vols, 1790–4).

Woodville, W., *The History of the Inoculation of the Smallpox in Great Britain* (London: Phillips, 1796).

Woodville, W., *Reports of a Series of Inoculations for the Variolae Vaccinae or Cow-pox* (London: Phillips, 1799).

Woodville, W., *Observations on the Cow-pox* (London: Phillips, 1800).

Zwanenberg, D. van, The Suttons and the business of inoculation, *Med. Hist.*, 1978, **22**, 71–82.

Index

ADAMS, J., 68, 150–2
Aikin, C. R., 184, 188
Alastrim, 15 (*see* smallpox)
Anderson, E. K., 182
Andre, Dr, 128
Angina pectoris, 41–2
Archard, L. C., 112, 185, 193
Arita, I., 10, 158, 194
Attenuation of smallpox, 8, 21–36,
   111–13, 127, 150–64, 184

BADCOCK, J., 156, 161, 163, 180
Baker, Sir G., 26, 73
Baker, J., 60, 79
Ballhorn, G. F., 80, 188–9
Banks, Sir J., 40, 44, 54, 91
Baron, J., 38, 84, 174, 196
   Jenner Biography, 38, 70, 129, 132,
      133, 174, 180
   Jenner's letters, 71, 75, 82, 91, 94,
      118, 130, 132, 145, 176, 177
Barry, F. W., 14
Bauer, D. J., 18
Bedson, Prof. H. S., 4, 112–13, 162,
   163, 185
Bevan, E., 143
Bishop, W. J., 31
Blandford, Dorset, 27
Blaxall, F. R., 159, 165, 178
Bollinger, O. von, 193
Bousquet, M., 181, 189, 191
Bovine herpes mammillitis, 137, 139,
   168
Boylston, Z., 21

Bradley, T., 143
Bristol University, 136–7, 141
Bulloch, Prof. W., 86–7
Bumpus, A., 8, 92, 105–17, 120, 128,
   185
Bumpus vaccine, 9, 93, 97–100, 129,
   131, 180, 195
Butcher, S., 93, 103, 106, 107, 115
Byles, J. B., 16

CARRO, J. DE, 133, 175–7, 195
Catlin, 13
Ceely, R., 138
   studies cowpox, 169–73, 180, 189
   variolates cows, 155–6, 161, 163
Chandler, B., 73
Chauveau, A., 159–60
Chickenpox (varicella), 17, 18, 19, 28,
   116, 143, 145
Christie, A. B., 34, 116, 126–7
Christie, T., 133
'Cigar-pox', 75, 104
Cline, H., 40, 53, 70
Colborne, Rev., 87–8
Collingridge, J., 105–6, 115
Cologne vaccine, 182
Condamine, C. M. de la, 25, 35
Contamination of vaccine,
   by bacteria, 71, 79, 83, 126, 138–40,
      146–8
   by viruses, 94, 98–104, 107–11, 130,
      152, 155–8, 162–3
Cook, Capt., 40
Cooke, C., 71

Copeman, S. A. M., 154, 156–9, 160, 163, 170
Cowpox, 2–4, 67, 136–7, 165–73, 170
  and smallpox, 67–8, 84–5
  as possible source of vaccinia, 4, 107–11, 185–91
  in nineteenth century, 168–73, 187–91
  Jenner's cases, 55–9, 67
  repeat attacks of, 66, 76–8
  safety of, 67, 78–9, 188–90
  severity of, 67–8, 71, 78–88, 96–7, 146–9, 166–7, 187–91
  variolation compared with, 67–8, 79–85
Creaser, T., 129
Creighton, C., 8, 79, 86–7, 132–3, 154, 190, 191
  criticizes Jenner, 38, 45–6, 49–50, 79, 84–5, 134, 136, 195
  on cowpox, 74–5, 84–5, 103–4, 132–3, 142, 191
  on spurious cowpox, 78, 134, 136, 142, 148
  variolous test, 72–3, 74–5
Crookshank, E. M., 8, 37, 50, 54, 79, 85–6, 133–6, 154, 163, 181
  on cowpox, 77, 82–3, 102–3, 147–9, 163, 169–70, 171–3, 177, 191
  on spurious cowpox, 135–6
  subjective views of, 82–3, 86, 135–6, 147–9, 187, 190
Crummer, L. R., 46
Cuckoo, nesting habits, 42–6

DEKKING, F., ix, 191
Dick, Prof. G., 15
Dimsdale, Baron T., 27, 30–2, 33–4, 73
Dixon, Prof. C. W.,
  on Jenner, 39, 47, 119, 134, 141
  on smallpox, 11, 16, 28, 115–16
  on variolation, 21, 23, 30, 34, 36
Downie, Prof. A. W., 3, 4, 16, 28, 165, 191
Drewitt, F. D., 39, 46
Dudgeon, Prof. J. A., 179, 182
Dumbell, Prof. K. R., 4, 112–13, 162, 163, 185
Dunning, R., xiii, 132

EAUX AUX JAMBES, 177 (see also grease)
Ecuador vaccine, 182

EM63 vaccine, 182
Emetic tartar, 41, 49
Emond, R. T. D., 83–4, 190
English Royal Family, 12–13, 23
Equine coital exanthem, 178
Equine vaccine, see grease, horsepox, vaccinia
Eruptions after vaccination, 94–5, 97–101, 121–4
Esposito, J. J., 112, 185
Estlin, J. B., 181, 189, 190
Evans, J., 123, 130, 145
Excell, H., 62, 68, 80

FENNER, F., vi–viii, 11, 182, 193
Finch, Rev. W., 125–6
Fisk, D., 39
Foege, W. H., 18, 28
Fraser, H., 76
Frewen, Mr, 35

GARDNER, E., 52, 118
Gassner, Dr, 154
General inoculation, 31
Generalized vaccinia, 107, 114, 116
Gibbs, E. P. J., 136–9, 167, 171–2
Gins, H. A., 159
Gispen, R., 112
Gloucester Medical Society, 46, 53
Grease, 64–6, 75–6, 141–2, 171–8, 192–5
Greenwood, M., 39, 48
Gregory, G., 146, 181
Grosvenor, Hon. R., 144
Guarnieri, G., 193
Guillou, F.-A., 152–3

HARRISON, Dr, 124
Harper, L., 112
Haygarth, J., 12, 27, 28–9, 32, 33, 35, 53, 129, 196
Heberden, W., 27, 42
Hellman, C. D., 46
Henderson, D. A., 10, 18, 28, 158
Herrlich, Prof. A., 154, 161, 192
Hickes, J., 46, 53
Hicks, H., 97, 100, 105, 114
Hime, T. W., 109–10, 157, 161, 163
Holt, Rev. R., 124, 189
Home, E., 40, 42, 53, 54
Hopkins, D., 11
Horgan, E. S., 4, 158–9, 161
Horsepox, 170, 174–8, 192–5

Houlton, Rev. R., 26
Hughes, T., 87–8, 148
Hungerford, T. G., 178
Hunter, J., 39–44, 47–9, 53
Hutchinson, J. R., 179, 180
Hybrids, 4, 113–14, 123, 130, 185, 191

INGENHOUSZ, J., 70–1, 134, 140

JENNER E., 1, 2, 6–8, 37, 118–19, 130,
    150, 179–80
  career and character, 38–51, 118–19,
    195–6
  cowpox, 56, 67, 99, 169
  eruptions caused by vaccine, 97–8,
    101, 128
  grease, 64–6, 75–6, 141–2, 171–6, 180
  Inquiry analysed, 68–88
  Inquiry described, 52–67
  spurious cowpox, 66–7, 78, 134–49
  vaccines, 59–63, 87, 97, 125, 131, 146,
    188
  variolous test, 56, 63, 74
Jenner, G., 7
Jenner, H., 43, 58, 63–4, 74
Jenner, S., 97, 130
Jesty, B., 37, 86

KAPLAN, Prof. C., 182
Kelsch, L. F. A., 160
Kelson, T. M., 122, 152
Kentish Town vaccine, 99–100, 129,
    131, 142, 180
Kirtland, G., 80, 189–90
Kirkpatrick, J., 23
Klein, E., 157–8, 163

LAFONT, Dr, 132, 176, 192
Lauder, I. M., 171
Lawrence, J., 82
Le Fanu, W. R., 39, 46
Lettsom, John C., 31, 44, 148
Lister Institute vaccine, 182
Loy, J., 174–6, 192
Ludlow, D., 39, 52, 56

MACAULAY, BARON T., 14
Mackett, M., 112, 185, 193
Maitland, C., 22–3, 30
Maladie du coït, 177–8
Marblehead, Mass., 127–9
Marennikova, S. S., 193

Marshall, J., 99–100, 105, 114, 131
Marson, Mr, 181, 189, 190
Martin, W. B., 137
Martindale's Pharmacopoeia, 41
Massachusetts vaccine, 182
Mather, Rev. C., 21
Mayr, Prof. A., 192
McConnell, S. J., 158
McVail, J. C., 6, 104, 108, 184, 189–90
Melon, Mr, 177
Miller, G., 21, 22, 23, 25, 36
Mitchell, Dr, 124
Monkeypox, 158, 193, 194
Monro, A., 144–5, 176
Montagu, Lady Mary Wortley, 22
Moore J., 27, 176, 179
Moseley B., 85
Mutants 4, 35–6, 111–13, 161–2, 185–7,
    193

NATIONAL VACCINE
    ESTABLISHMENT, 51, 131,
    144, 176, 179–80
Nelmes, S., 58, 82, 189
New York Board of Health, 182
Nizamuddin, M., 112
Noehden, A. A., 132

O'MALLEY, J., 37
Osborne, A. D., 141, 167

PADDINGTON COWPOX, 120, 128
Paget, Sir J., 54
Parry, C., 42, 46, 68
Pasteur, L., 2, 86, 196
Paul, H., 14
Paytherus, T., 46, 80, 101, 147–8
Pead, W., 60–2, 63, 74
Pearlpox, 151
Pearson, G., 5, 37, 50–1, 53, 55, 91, 105,
    118–19, 135, 185, 188–9, 195
  his Inquiry, 71–2, 75–9, 118, 193
  severity of cowpox, 82, 123–4, 189
  threads, 97, 118–32, 152
  variolation, 27, 36
  views on eruptions, 94, 97–8, 128
Petworth, Sussex, 127–8
Phipps, J., 52, 54, 58–9
Plague, 13–14
Pseudocowpox, 137, 139, 166–7
Pustules following vaccination, 94,
    97–9, 121–3
Pylarini, J., 22

RANBY, J., 25, 27, 35
Rao, A. R., 19
Rashes following vaccination, 124–7
Razzell, P. E.,
    attenuation of smallpox, 4, 8, 104,
        111, 133, 184
    severity of vaccination, 127, 128, 129
    variolation, 24, 32, 153
Redfearn, R., 121–2, 130
Rhazes, 11
Ricketts, T. F., 16
Ring, J., 98, 102, 120, 125, 132–3
Ringer, S., 41
Rosenwald, C. D., 24
Roseola vaccina, 126
Roseola variolosa, 126
Royal Commission (1898), 6, 73, 74,
    103, 104, 108, 131–2, 133, 159–60
Ruston, T., 34

SACCO, L., 132–3, 142, 171, 176,
    192–3, 195
Sainsbury, H., 41
Sanfelice, F., 193
Saunders, P., 47
Simon, Sir J., 6, 13, 52
Sims, J., 71, 82
Smadel, J., 190
Smallpox
    after vaccination, 142–6
    and cowpox, 66–8, 80–2, 134–49, 170
    Ann Bumpus, 107–14
    attenuation, 21–36, 111–13, 150–5
    caused by vaccination, 121–4, 127–9
    clinical features and history, 10–20
    communicability, 28–33
    in animals, 154–64
    source of vaccinia, 102–3, 111–13,
        150–64, 184–5, 192
Smallpox Hospital, London, 5, 30, 89
Spontaneous cowpox, 67, 142, 170
Spots after vaccination, 124–7
Spurious cowpox, 66–7, 78, 134–49,
    168, 196
    grease, 141–2
    Jenner's categories, 135, 138, 140,
        141
    smallpox after, 71, 142–6
Stearn, E. W., and A. E., 13
Stevenson, J., 143–4
Stinchcomb, W., 57, 81–2
Stonehouse vaccine, 87–8, 148, 187
Story, E., 129

Stromeyer, C., 80, 125, 188–9
Sutton, D., 25–7, 30, 33, 73
Swinepox, 53, 151
Syphilis, 1, 85, 103
TANNER, T., 91, 131, 174, 180
Teissier, P., 160
Theile, B., 153, 154–6
Thomson, J., 145
Thornton, E., 88, 148
Timoni, E., 22
Transformation, 111–12, 161–3, 193–5
Travers, B., 49
Trousseau, Prof. A., 153–4
True cowpox, 134–49
Turner, A., 185

ULCERATION IN COWPOX, 67, 71,
    79–88, 146–9
Underwood, E. A., 129

VACCINATION, 16, 19, 24, 73–4, 116
Vaccination Act (1840), 14, 179
Vaccination Act (1898), 180
Vaccines
    Bumpus, 97, 107–14, 131
    compared, 180–95
    equine, 142, 175–8, 180
    eruptions, 94, 97–101, 121–4
    Jenner's, 59–64, 87
    modern, 83–4, 119–20, 182–3
    Pearson's threads, 118–31
    Woodville's, 91–6, 102–4, 115–17
Vaccinia
    from cowpox, 4, 108–11, 142, 165–6,
        185–91, 193–4
    from horsepox, 4, 142, 177–8, 192–3
    from hybrids, 4, 113–14, 123, 185
    from smallpox, 4, 35–6, 109–13,
        150–64, 184–5, 193–4
    not found naturally, 3, 137, 165–6
    origins, 4–9, 102–4, 179–95
Variola major, 11, 15, 35
Variola minor (alastrim), 15, 35
Variolation, 8,
    after Jenner, 150–64
    before Jenner, 21–37
    communicability, 28–33
    compared with cowpox, 67–8, 79–85,
        95
    mortality, 24–7
    of animals, 154–64
    source of vaccinia, 36, 111, 150–64
'Varioloid', 145–6, 152

Variolous test, 56, 63–4, 72–5
Viborg, E., 154

WARD, M., 122–3
Warts, 137
Waterhouse, B., 48, 129, 132
Wehrle, P. F., 28
Whyte, D., 133
Willan, R., 27, 91 108–9, 113–14, 126,
    142–3, 189
Williams, G., 165
Winslow, O. E., 21

Winterburn, G. W., 156
Woodville, W., 5–9, 55, 68, 72, 75,
    89–91, 119, 184, 188, 195
  Bumpus, 92, 97, 105–7, 185
  eruptions from vaccine, 94–5, 99–100
  Observations, 99–101
  on variolation, 25, 26, 27, 30, 34, 35,
    80, 95
  origins of his vaccines, 102–4, 114
  Reports, 91–4, 120

ZWANNENBERG, D. VAN, 26